The Secrets of Great

G SPOT ORGASMS
AND FEMALE EJACULATION

THE *best* POSITIONS AND LATEST TECHNIQUES FOR
CREATING *powerful, long-lasting, full-body* ORGASMS

TRISTAN TAORMINO

QUIVER

© 2011 Quiver
Text © 2011 Tristan Taormino
Photography © 2011 Quiver

First published in the USA in 2011 by
Quiver, a member of
Quayside Publishing Group
100 Cummings Center
Suite 406-L
Beverly, MA 01915-6101
www.quiverbooks.com

The Publisher maintains the records relating to images in this book required by 18 USC 2257. Records are located at Rockport Publishers, Inc., 100 Cummings Center, Suite 406-L, Beverly, MA 01915-6101.

13 12   2 3 4 5

ISBN-13: 978-1-59233-456-8
ISBN-10: 1-59233-456-3

Digital edition published in 2012

Library of Congress Cataloging-in-Publication Data available

"The ABGs" © 2010 by Alison Tyler
"Girl Talk" © 2010 by Rachel Kramer Bussel
"Fly" © 2008 by Valerie Alexander, first appeared in
Best Women's Erotica 2009, edited by Violet Blue (San Francisco: Cleis Press, 2008)

Anatomical drawings © 2010 by Katie Diamond and Tristan Taormino Enterprises, Inc.
Book design by Traffic Design Consultants Ltd.
Photography by Holly Randall Photography

Printed and bound in Singapore

CONTENTS

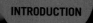

LET YOUR G-SPOT ADVENTURE BEGIN

I've been writing and teaching about sex for fifteen years, and during that time, I've taught hundreds of workshops around the world to all different kinds of people. Sometimes, I have the pleasure of leading a hands-on class in which I lecture first, and then participants get to try out techniques. I once taught a G-spot class to fifty couples at a private event. After I explained about anatomy, arousal, stimulation techniques, positions, and female ejaculation, they were free to explore.

One woman asked me, "Is it possible that I just don't have a G-spot? I've looked and can't find it!" I worked with her and her partner, who confessed he wasn't sure what to do. He slid his fingers inside her vagina, and I talked him through until he found it. I encouraged him to apply more pressure to the area, and suddenly she squeeled, "Oh! That's it!" Later that evening, she approached me and said, "We've been together for fifteen years. After your workshop, we went back to our room, and I had a totally different kind of orgasm. It was amazing! You've changed my sex life!" I treasure those experiences in which I get to make a real difference in people's erotic lives.

In recent articles about the G-spot, *Cosmopolitan Magazine* raved "Have Your Best Orgasm!" *Men's Health* promised "Be Her Best Ever!" and *Playboy* touted "Female Orgasm Mysteries Revealed!" If you got all your sexual information from magazine headlines, you'd think the G-spot were some kind of holy grail, the answer to all your sexual questions and then some. I'm going to burst your bubble: It's not. Too often, especially in mainstream media, the G-spot has been positioned as trendy, hip, and the key to the best sex of your life. It isn't.

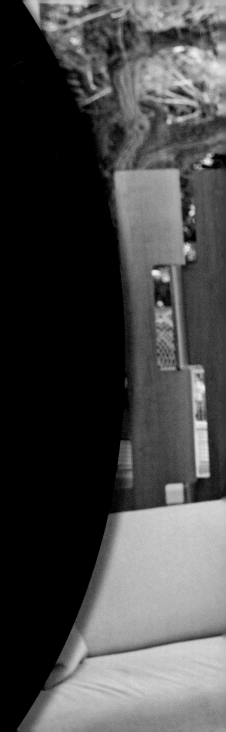

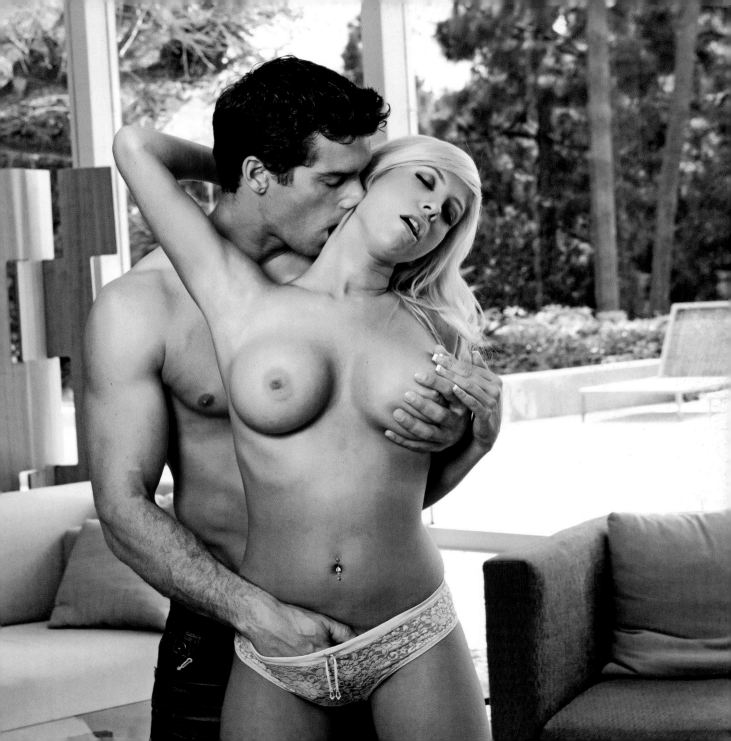

The workshops I teach and this book don't perpetuate that illusion. I wrote this book to educate by providing real, useful information. I did it to validate women's experiences and help them better understand their bodies. I did it to open women up to all the diverse possibilities of pleasure at their fingertips.

One of the important accomplishments of Alice Kahn Ladas, Beverly Whipple, and John Perry, authors of The G-Spot, was that they gave a name to this pleasure center. Naming it helped demystify it and support women's own sexual experiences. I'll talk more about how the G-spot got its name and some of the controversies surrounding it in chapter 1; in chapter 2, I'll give you a road map to help you visualize female sexual anatomy and how the G-spot fits in. Learning about the G-spot—what it is, where it is, how it works, and what it can do—is the first step toward a better understanding of our bodies and the potential for erotic enjoyment they hold. This knowledge contributes to broadening our ideas about erogenous zones, pleasure, and sexual satisfaction. It can support some of the feelings and experiences you've already had.

At another one of my workshops, a woman told me that nearly every one of her orgasms had come from clitoral stimulation. It could be oral sex, rubbing with her hand, or using a vibrator, but, as she said, "My clit always has to be in the mix." Then she told a story about how once she was masturbating with an insertable vibrator and she came without stimulating her clitoris. "I don't know if it was the toy, a certain angle, or what. I don't remember what was so different that time. It was such an intense feeling, and I want to know how to experience it again!"

Hers is a story I've heard from plenty of women. They seemingly "stumble" on a new kind of orgasm after being dedicated clit girls for years, but they're not sure how to replicate it. There's a good chance these women had G-spot orgasms. In fact, when women learn more about their G-spots and try different stimulation techniques, they discover they can make it happen again. Chapters 3 and 6 will give you pointers about arousal and G-spot exploration. And speaking of sex toys, find out about the best kinds for the G-spot in chapter 4.

Educating yourself about the G-spot can help illuminate a new area of your sexuality to explore. Learning how to target this sensitive area can bring you something new to enjoy during masturbation and partnered sex. As you try different techniques, positions, and toys, you'll find out what works for you. That information can help connect you and your partner and enhance your sexual relationship. Find out more about G-spot stimulation during partnered sex (including the connection between the G-spot and anal sex) in chapters 6, 7, and 8.

Plenty of women find that having an orgasm during vaginal intercourse is a challenge. Dr. Elisabeth Lloyd, professor of biology at Indiana University and author of The Case of the Female Orgasm: Bias in the Science of Evolution, analyzed thirty-two studies, conducted over a period of seventy-four years, of the frequency of female orgasm during intercourse. She concluded that when intercourse did not include clitoral stimulation, only a quarter of the women studied experienced orgasms often or very often during intercourse.[1] Plenty of other studies back up Dr. Lloyd's. If you enjoy penetration and want to be able to climax from it, learning about your G-spot is an important piece of the puzzle. For many women, trying positions that offer access to the G-spot and concentrate stimulation on the G-spot can increase your chances of an orgasm during intercourse with your partner.

Some women say that a G-spot orgasm is one of several types of orgasms they experience and it definitely feels distinct from other types. Some report it provides a deeper, all-over body feeling than a clitoral orgasm does. Others describe it as a powerful release that resonates throughout their bodies, not just between their legs. Still others assert that their G-spot orgasms last longer than other orgasms. And, yes, some women say it's the best orgasm of their lives. G-spot orgasms are possible, desirable, and even preferable for some (but not all) women. Read more about these types of orgasms—and how to increase your chances of having one—in chapter 10.

Don't think of G-spot orgasms in terms of better or worse, longer or shorter, easier or more difficult. Instead, think of them as unique, individual, and FUN! Remember, this is all about pleasure, so don't get caught up in definitions and hierarchies. Your experience is your experience.

Deborah Sundahl, a sex education pioneer and author of *Female Ejaculation and the G-Spot*, describes the G-spot as a kind of gateway to sexual evolution and points out that unlocking the secrets of the G-spot can also bring you closer to female ejaculation. Whether you're an experienced ejaculator, you've ejaculated before but aren't sure how to do it again, or you're interested in learning how, knowing about your G-spot is the first step toward enjoying this unique activity. In most cases, you have to master your G-spot before you can ejaculate. In chapters 11 and 12, you'll find out all you ever wanted to know about female ejaculation and squirting orgasms.

Throughout this book, I've included erotic stories that feature G-spot stimulation, written by three amazingly talented writers: Alison Tyler, Rachel Kramer Bussel, and Valerie Alexander. I hope they'll inspire you in a different way to explore the world of the G-spot.

As you read this book, keep an open mind about what you can learn from it. Although I often use male/female pronouns for consistency throughout the text, please know that the information applies to anyone of any gender and sexual orientation who has a G-spot or whose partner has a G-spot. I hope *The Secrets of Great G-Spot Orgasms and Female Ejaculation* gives you plenty of ideas and inspires new exploration. I hope you gain a greater understanding of your body, a new way to experience pleasure, techniques for enhancing sex with yourself and a partner, and more orgasmic possibilities.

Remember, don't pressure yourself to love G-spot sex if you don't. Be willing, though, to give it a try. You might just find a pleasant surprise at the other end of the adventure!

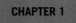

CHAPTER 1

DOES IT EXIST? A HISTORY OF THE G-SPOT AND THE GREAT DEBATE

My explorations . . . have shown me the G-spot's unique ability to enhance not only women's physical pleasure but also their intimate relationships with themselves and others. The idea that female sexuality is not simple, but evolves and expands throughout one's lifetime is an enticing promise. And at the heart of this idea—and at the heart of women's sexual evolution—dwells female ejaculation and its source, the G-spot.

—Deborah Sundahl[2]

Women's sexuality has a long history of being discounted, misunderstood, misrepresented, medicalized, or left out of the picture (and research studies and textbooks) altogether. Beginning in the late 1800s, vaginal intercourse was lauded as the best way for women to experience pleasure and orgasm, yet little was known about how or why.

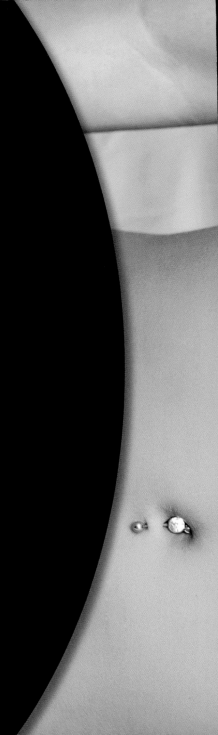

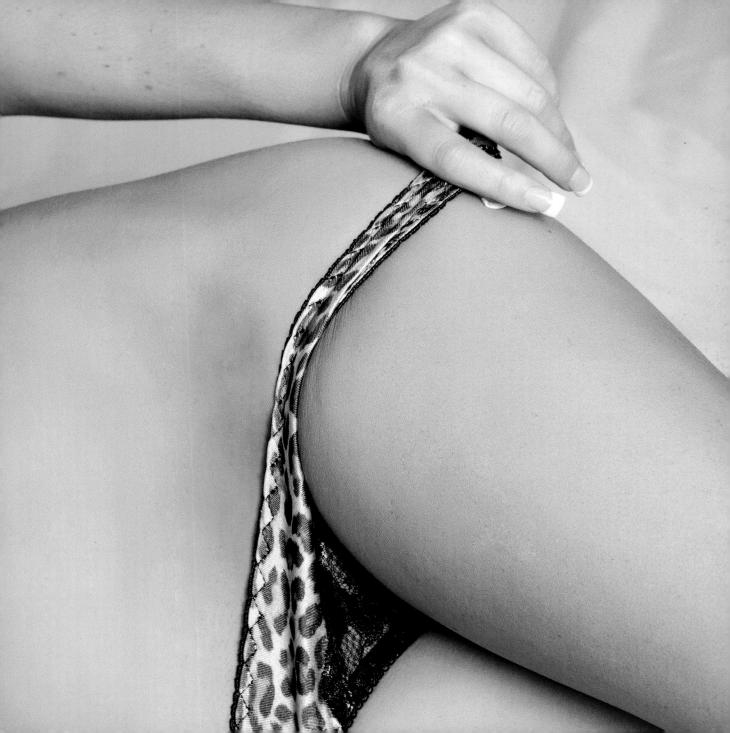

A BRIEF HISTORY OF THE G-SPOT

A German gynecologist named Ernest Grafenberg first wrote about what we now call the G-spot. In 1950, Grafenberg published a paper about sexual satisfaction and orgasm in women. In "The Role of Urethra in Female Orgasm," he identified a sensitive area in the front of the vagina near the pubic bone. He referred to the urethra as being surrounded by erectile tissue and said the area swelled during stimulation. He also observed that some women expelled fluid from the urethra at the moment of orgasm, and the fluid was not urine. He even talked about how position and angle were crucial for stimulating the spot—apparently, he was a fan of Doggie Style, which topped the list for best positions. At the time, his findings were controversial amid a growing debate over whether women had vaginal or clitoral orgasms.

When Alfred Kinsey released his book *Sexual Behavior in the Human Female* in 1953, everything changed. The book was based on a widespread study of female sexual desire, behavior, and orgasm. From it, Kinsey concluded that the clitoris, not the vagina, was the central pleasure receptor for women. Then came famed researchers Masters and Johnson. In their 1966 book *Human Sexual Response*, they argued that the clitoris extended beyond the clitoral glans and shaft and included several different structures behind the labia. They concluded that all female orgasms—including those that occurred through intercourse alone—were therefore clitoral orgasms.

Around the same time, the women's movement was gaining momentum. Women began consciousness-raising groups in which they talked openly with each other about what really got them off. Their focus on the clitoris gave them sexual autonomy and empowerment. They challenged an intercourse-centric view of pleasure as an extension of sexism and the patriarchy. The clitoris become the center of attention, which was great on one level, but it also told women who enjoyed other kinds of stimulation that they weren't in the norm—and it didn't tell the whole story about female sexuality.

In 1980, *The G-Spot: And Other Discoveries About Human Sexuality* by Alice Kahn Ladas, Beverly Whipple, and John D. Perry was published and quickly became a best seller. Based on their original research study of 400 women, the authors identified an area located inside and on the front wall of the vagina that was very sensitive to deep pressure. They named it the Grafenberg Spot in honor of Ernest Grafenberg, and nicknamed it the G-spot.

Ladas, Whipple, and Perry wrote that the G-spot felt like a small bean, and, when a woman was aroused, it could swell to the size of a dime or even a half-dollar. In order to explain why others before them hadn't noted it and why women may not have found it themselves, they posited that when a woman was not yet aroused, the G-spot was difficult if not impossible to find. Likened to an area called the urethral sponge (a term coined by the authors in the Federation of Feminist Women's Health Centers who wrote *A New View of a Woman's Body*), the G-spot was described as "probably composed of a complex network of blood vessels, the paraurethral glands and ducts (female prostate), nerve endings, and the tissue surrounding the urethral neck."[3] The authors of *A New View of a Woman's Body* argued that the G-spot was a significant part of female pleasure and orgasm.

During the 1980s and '90s, no significant research emerged to support or refute the claims of Ladas, Whipple, and Perry. While some sexologists and scientists applauded *The G-Spot* and others denounced it, the mainstream media embraced the book and its findings with gusto. Women's magazines featured article after article about how to find the magic spot. Adult novelty companies marketed toys designed to hit the spot, and women everywhere were looking for the spot. As the G-spot seeped into popular consciousness, more women began to explore their bodies and discover that all this talk about the G-spot really resonated with their own sexual experiences. This all culminated in a veritable G-spot frenzy in the '90s that continued into the next decade, when G-spot books, toys, workshops, and videos became a central part of female-driven adult sex education.

THE GREAT G-SPOT DEBATE

Debates began within academic and scientific communities about the existence of the G-spot and its role in female pleasure. One of the first studies to receive a lot of mainstream press was Terence Hines's 2001 opinion piece published in the *American Journal of Obstetrics & Gynecology*. Hines's essay was a cursory look at the literature about the G-spot and his *opinion* about whether there was enough scientific evidence to support its existence; in it, he famously called the G-spot "a gynecological UFO." This sparked worldwide speculation that the G-spot did not exist.

EVERYTHING'S CONNECTED

That came on the heels of Rebecca Chalker's pivotal book *The Clitoral Truth*, in which Chalker argued that the urethral sponge is part of the clitoris, so any orgasm that comes from stimulating the sponge is still a clitoral orgasm. Likewise, in her 2006 article "Anatomy of the Clitoris," Helen O'Connell, M.D., head of neurology at the Royal Melbourne Hospital in Australia, agreed that the vaginal wall was part of the clitoris. She said the triangular walls of the clitoris wrapped around the urethra and were composed of erectile tissue that becomes engorged during arousal. These works technically refuted the G-spot; however, it was more a matter of semantics. They clearly supported the idea of the urethral sponge made of erectile tissue and a sensitive area on the front wall of the vagina—they just reframed it with different language.

A 2008 study at Italy's University of L'Aquila took a new approach to the subject. Researchers asked twenty women how they achieved orgasm, and then took ultrasound scans of their bodies. Eleven women told researchers they had never had an orgasm from vaginal penetration alone. The other nine women said they did have orgasms from vaginal penetration without clitoral or other stimulation. The ultrasounds of this second group revealed that these women had thicker tissue on or near the urethral sponge than the first group.[4] One could conclude that the women with more pronounced urethral sponges had an easier time finding the G-spot or showing their partners how to find it and, therefore, were more likely to experience a G-spot orgasm. Critics said no conclusions could be made about any of it because the sample of the study was so small.

In 2010, scientists at King's College in London published their findings from a study done the year before. The article got a lot of attention in the mainstream press because the sample size was quite large: More than 1,800 women who were all identical or fraternal twins participated. Headlines read: "New Study Says G-spot Doesn't Exist," "What an Anti-Climax: G-spot Is a Myth," "There's No G-spot So Stop Looking for It," and "G-spot Is a Figment of Imagination." The articles then "summarized" the researchers' claim that there was no physiological basis for the G-spot. Most of the reporters hadn't read the actual article, but culled together the most "newsworthy" points from the abstract and the press release.

Critics fired back that both the study methods and the reporting about it were flawed. For example, the study was based entirely on interviews with the subjects. Women were asked pointed questions such as, "Do you believe you have a so-called G-spot, a small area the size of a 20p coin on the front wall of your vagina that is sensitive to deep pressure?"[5] Researchers did not describe or define the G-spot any further; therefore, women who'd never heard of the G-spot or who'd never found or explored their G-spots would likely say no. Interestingly, none of the reporters pointed out that 56 percent of the women answered yes to that question.

DOES SHE OR DOESN'T SHE?

Between 63 and 71 percent of the women in the King's College study said it was "not difficult at all" for them to have an orgasm through clitoral stimulation. When asked to rate the ease or difficulty of having a vaginal orgasm, 40 to 48 percent ranked it "not difficult at all." Because of this difference the King's College researchers concluded, "The hypothetical G-spot is neither necessary nor sufficient for a woman to experience a vaginal orgasm, providing legitimate grounds to further question its existence."

But what about that 40 to 48 percent who found it easy to have an orgasm from vaginal stimulation? Plenty of interesting details were also glossed over in the media coverage. For example, women who were more orgasmic were more likely to say they had a G-spot. Women who felt more fulfilled in their relationships, along with younger women, were more likely to say they had a G-spot. The women who reported they did have a G-spot also reported that they were more satisfied with their sex partners.[6]

Less than a month later, gynecologists gathered in Paris for "G-Day," a conference organized by French gynecologist Sylvain Mimoun to dispute the British study. About the study, Mimoun pointed out that women can only say they have a G-spot if they've found and explored it. "In discovering the sensitive parts of her own body, this sensitive zone [the G-spot] will become more and more functional. But if she has never touched it and no one else has ever touched it . . . it won't exist for her as a consequence."[7]

SO WHERE DOES THAT LEAVE US?

Substantial research into female anatomy and sexuality during the past sixty years has added to our knowledge about women, sex, and satisfaction. We have a much more complex view of female anatomy, desire, and pleasure today, and that's a good thing. However, when it comes to the G-spot and female ejaculation, we need more research, especially studies that are anatomically based, include women of all sexual orientations, take a broader view on sexual history and experience, and focus on stimulation methods other than just intercourse.

For all the women who answered yes to that British survey question, the hundreds interviewed for *The G-Spot*, and the thousands I've talked to in my fifteen-year career as a sex educator, the G-spot definitely exists. And although it's very sensitive, it doesn't care what its critics say about it.

CHAPTER 2

WHERE IS IT? A ROAD MAP FOR FINDING THE G-SPOT

When my G-spot is hit, it's like a flood of emotion with a release that makes me feel free. Stress melts away and that feeling fills my head with thoughts of flying in the softest clouds. Like I'm free from all my worries right then and there. I guess I just have a fantastic partner.

—Roxie

To better understand the G-spot, where it is, and what it does, we must first look at female sexuality as a whole. The female genitals are often reduced to a schoolyard distinction: He has a penis, and she has a vagina. Actually, a woman has a vulva, and the vagina is one part of it, but she also has plenty more significant parts that play a big role in sexual stimulation and satisfaction. Learning where different structures are, what they do, and how they affect each other is the first step toward discovering the G-spot.

GETTING TO KNOW YOUR ANATOMY

To better understand how the G-spot is connected to female pleasure, let's look at female sexual anatomy as a whole, inside and out. The vulva encompasses all the external parts of the female genitals, including the inner and outer labia, the clitoral hood and glans, the pubic mound, the vaginal opening, and the urethral opening. We'll also look at the anus and PC muscles.

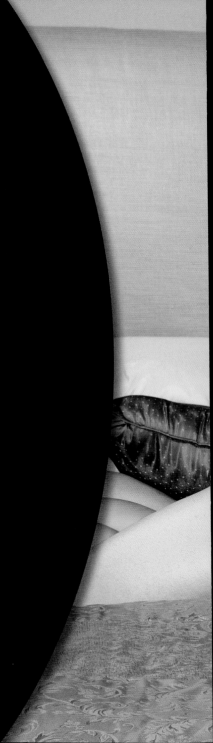

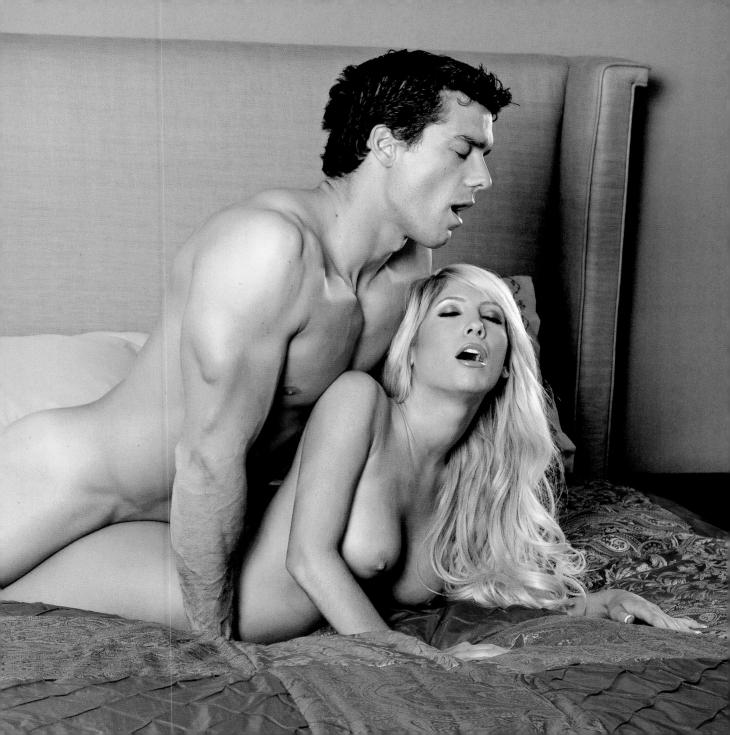

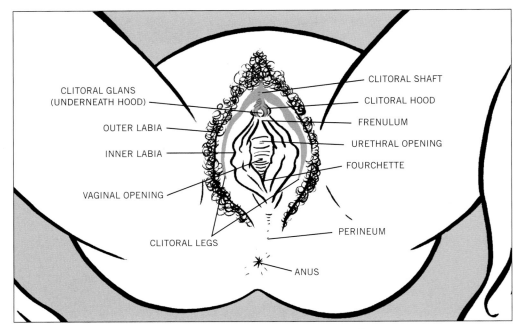

CLITORAL GLANS
(UNDERNEATH HOOD)

CLITORAL SHAFT

CLITORAL HOOD

FRENULUM

OUTER LABIA

INNER LABIA

URETHRAL OPENING

FOURCHETTE

VAGINAL OPENING

PERINEUM

CLITORAL LEGS

ANUS

SHADED AREAS DENOTE INTERNAL PARTS.

THE LABIA

The outer labia (also know as labia majora) are the fleshy outer lips of the vulva on which pubic hair grows. The inner labia (or labia minora) are the inner lips of the vulva; these lips are smooth and hairless and contain lots of nerve endings, making them very sensitive to touch and stimulation. When a woman is aroused, the inner labia swell and deepen in color.

The inner labia may curve inward or flare outward and may be thin and narrow, thick and wide, or both. Most women have some kind of asymmetry in the appearance of their labia. Every woman's vulva is unique. Some have large outer labia and thin inner labia, some have thick inner labia and small outer labia—there are hundreds of combinations and possibilities.

The pubic mound (sometimes called the mons pubis) is the hair-covered patch of skin and fatty tissue that covers and protects the pubic bone. The area where the inner lips meet at the top is called the frenulum. Just above the frenulum is the clitoral hood, a tiny flap of skin that protects the clitoral glans.

THE CLITORAL STRUCTURE

The clitoral glans is what many people refer to simply as the clitoris, but it is actually just one (very supercharged) part of the clitoral structure. The clitoral glans is the most sensitive part of the clitoral structure (and of the entire human body); it contains 6,000 to 8,000 nerve endings, and its sole purpose is to act as a pleasure receptor. The glans is the external part of the clitoral shaft, which extends several inches back inside the body. The shaft splits into the legs of the clitoris that come down on either side behind the labia. Underneath the inner labia are also two bulbs of erectile tissue.

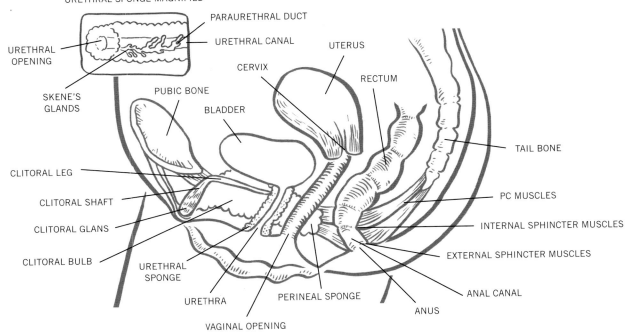

URETHRAL SPONGE MAGNIFIED
PARAURETHRAL DUCT
URETHRAL OPENING
URETHRAL CANAL
UTERUS
CERVIX
RECTUM
SKENE'S GLANDS
PUBIC BONE
BLADDER
TAIL BONE
CLITORAL LEG
CLITORAL SHAFT
CLITORAL GLANS
PC MUSCLES
INTERNAL SPHINCTER MUSCLES
EXTERNAL SPHINCTER MUSCLES
CLITORAL BULB
URETHRAL SPONGE
URETHRA
PERINEAL SPONGE
ANAL CANAL
ANUS
VAGINAL OPENING

When a woman is aroused, the glans retreats under the clitoral hood. The erectile tissue of the clitoral glans and shaft becomes engorged with blood and swells, and the glans and shaft become erect.

THE VAGINA

The vaginal opening is the entry to the vagina (also called the vaginal canal); at the inner end of the canal is the cervix. When a woman is aroused, the walls of the vagina begin to swell and produce lubrication. Depending on the woman, the inner two-thirds of the vagina or the entire canal and the opening expand, and the cervix and uterus move up.

It's important to note that a woman can be very aroused but her vagina may not lubricate enough to make penetration comfortable.

THE URETHRA

Just above the vaginal opening is the urethral opening, the external part of the urethra where urine exits the body. The urethra is the internal tube that leads to the bladder, and it is surrounded by spongy erectile tissue called the urethral sponge. It is sometimes referred to as the female prostate because of its similarities to the male prostate.

Part of the urethral sponge can be felt through the front wall of the vagina, about 1 to 2 inches (2.5 to 5 cm) inside the vaginal opening. This area on the front wall of the vagina, with the urethral sponge behind it, is known as the G-spot. When a woman is aroused, the erectile tissue of the urethral sponge gets engorged with blood, swells, and becomes more prominent. When the urethral sponge is erect, it becomes much more sensitive and many women find stimulation of it through the front wall of the vagina is very pleasurable. Keep in mind that the different structures of the clitoris—the shaft, legs, and bulb—are connected to the urethral sponge. In fact, some experts consider the urethral sponge to be a part of the clitoris. Thus, stimulation of the sponge activates the arousal of the clitoris, and vice versa.

The urethral sponge contains paraurethral glands and ducts; two of the thirty glands are called the Skene's glands, which are located very close to the opening of the urethra. During arousal, the Skene's glands (which are called the female prostate by some researchers) produce a fluid that is similar to the fluid produced by a man's prostate. The fluid can be released from the glands through paraurethral ducts into the urethra and out the body through the urethral opening. This is what's called female ejaculation, also known as vaginal ejaculation or squirting. (I'll talk more about female ejaculation in chapters 11 and 12.)

THE ANUS

Behind the vaginal opening is the perineum, a small but sensitive area. Behind the perineum is the anus, the opening to the anal canal and rectum, which is made of soft tissue that is rich in nerve endings. It has a puckered appearance, and the skin around it contains hair follicles.

Just inside the anus are the external and internal sphincter muscles. These muscles give the anus that tight feeling and also control bowel movements. We must learn to relax these muscles to achieve comfortable anal penetration.

Closer to the opening is the external sphincter. You can learn to control the external sphincter, making it tense or relaxed. The internal sphincter, on the other hand, is controlled by the autonomic nervous system, which also controls such involuntary body functions as breathing rate. This muscle ordinarily reacts reflexively; for example, when you are ready to have a bowel movement, the internal sphincter relaxes, allowing feces to move from the rectum to the anal canal and out the anus. The external and the internal sphincter muscles can work independently of each other, but because they overlap, they often work together. The more aware you are of your sphincters and the more you practice using them, the more toned they will be.

The first few inches inside the anus make up the anal canal, which is composed of soft, sensitive tissue with a high concentration of nerve endings. Beyond the anal canal is the rectum, which is about 8 or 9 inches (20 to 23 cm) long and made up of folds of soft, smooth tissue. When you are aroused, the rectum has the ability expand, which makes penetration possible.

THE PC MUSCLES

At the bottom of the pelvic floor is a group of broad, flat muscles called the pubococcygeus (pronounced *pew-bo-cock-se-gee-us*) muscles, or PC muscles for short. The urethra, vagina, and anus pass through these muscles, which support the pelvis from the pubic bone to the tailbone. To find your PC muscles, pretend that you're peeing and want to stop the flow of urine—the muscles you use are your PC muscles.

The PC muscles are an important part of sexual anatomy because they support the clitoral structure, vagina, and anus. Women who regularly exercise their PC muscle report many benefits, including better bladder control, more pleasurable penetration, better control of their orgasms, and stronger, longer orgasms.

KEEP AN OPEN MIND

The first step to great G-spot stimulation might surprise you: Keep an open mind. Pleasure doesn't just depend on good technique, a fantastic sex toy, or the perfect position. It's also about chemistry, communication, and feeling comfortable enough to shed your inhibitions. Your emotions and psychological state play a big role in your experience of sex.

Ideally, you can come to a sexual experience and ignore the rest of the world for the time being: Forget about the bills, the kids, the work schedule, and your other stressors. Let all of it just sit in the background while you bring your focus to your body, your partner, and your sexual connection. The more in touch you are with your body and the more sexually confident you feel, the better all kinds of sex will be.

REFRAMING FOREPLAY

A frequent complaint among women is that they don't get enough (or *any*) foreplay before intercourse. First, let me disclose my bias: I hate the word *foreplay* and the whole concept of it. For one, it positions all sorts of fabulous activities—including kissing, teasing, oral sex, manual stimulation, mutual masturbation, playing with sex toys—as merely appetizers before the main course. These activities are pleasurable and orgasmic for plenty of women and men, and I'm tired of them being considered only a side dish.

Foreplay makes intercourse the end goal, the ultimate conclusion, but shouldn't everyone's emphasis be on pleasure and enjoyment and (if you're lucky) orgasm? The formula of "foreplay, then intercourse," feels far too limiting. I know from talking to thousands of couples over the years that it just doesn't describe how they have sex. So, part of having an open mind is rethinking how we define sex and considering the myriad ways we can make ourselves and our partners feel good.

With all that said, I don't want to dismiss women's dissatisfaction with the lack of foreplay. This complaint is valid for many reasons and we need to listen to it. I'd like to reframe the idea, so that all women enjoy warming up to whatever kinds of activities come next. A woman's arousal cycle is as unique as she is, and it can change each time she has sex depending on her mood, the circumstances, her partner (if she has one), and lots of other factors.

However, the body still goes through a process during arousal, and most women need time to get to the point at which their bodies are ready for intense stimulation of all kinds. One of the things we know about the G-spot is that it's much easier to find when a woman is aroused, because it swells and becomes more prominent. We also know that once it swells, it's much more receptive to stimulation and that stimulation needs to be pretty vigorous. The lesson here is simple: You can't just hop on and soar into the heavens. You've got to warm up the engine first.

TURN HER ON BEFORE YOU TURN IT UP: AROUSAL

According to famed sexologists Masters and Johnson, who mapped the female arousal cycle in 1966, the cycle includes several phases. The first phase is the beginning of arousal, which Masters and Johnson called the excitement phase. Your heart rate and blood pressure both increase and you begin to breathe heavier. Blood flow increases to your genitals, beginning the engorgement process. This is when the outer labia move apart and the inner labia begin to swell; the vaginal walls lubricate, and the clitoral glans swells and becomes erect.

During this phase, you may feel sensations in your pelvic region as if all the blood is rushing to that one area, and you may feel dampness at the vaginal opening. The vagina expands, and the cervix and uterus move upward. Your nipples may also get erect and your skin may flush. You want to really savor this part of the arousal process and don't make any big moves—think slow and gentle. Your body is starting to come alive, so let this happen at its own pace. Remember, neither the clitoris nor the G-spot may be ready for stimulation at this point.

Next comes the plateau phase, during which the inner labia and clitoris continue to swell and the clitoral glans retreats under the clitoral hood. The inner labia changes color from pink to bright red or dark burgundy. During the plateau phase, the G-spot, the clitoral glans, and all the erectile tissue in the area are swollen. Your genitals are ready for and receptive to targeted stimulation.

Keep in mind that the phases are not necessarily clearly defined from one another—they may run into each other and are not the same every time you masturbate or have sex. In fact, subsequent research has shown that the cycle is quite variable in terms of how long each phase lasts. You can have a very long excitement phase as you work your way up to the plateau. You could get excited quickly, but have a longer plateau phase. Women who experience a long plateau phase can get frustrated or even give up on having an orgasm. But remember that each woman's experience of arousal is different. Knowing your body and your own unique rhythm is what's most important, rather than watching the clock (which is not conducive to an orgasm!). The plateau phase builds until you feel like you're on the edge of a cliff. If you make it over the edge, you experience orgasm, and then resolution.

EXERCISE: FINDING YOUR G-SPOT

1. Begin a masturbation session and tell yourself that you are under absolutely no pressure. Let go of expectations: No one is timing you and this is not a test! Remind yourself that this is a fact-finding mission, one that won't necessarily end in orgasm, and that's okay.

2. Start to explore your outer and inner labia with your hand. Use gentle strokes and let your body relax into the feelings.

3. Find some wetness at your vaginal opening, or use some of your favorite lube, and spread it around your labia, massaging the labia as you do.

4. When you're ready, begin to stimulate the areas around your clitoris. You can rub above the clitoral hood, on either side of it, or just below it. The idea is to tease yourself, which will help build arousal.

5. When you feel ready, slip a well-lubed finger inside your vaginal opening with one hand, while continuing to tease around your clit with the other. When you want to, edge toward the clitoral hood and stimulate the hood.

6. Slide your middle finger inside your vagina. Begin to slide it in and out. Add another finger if you want. Keep up the clitoral stimulation with your other hand, or if that's too awkward (or you prefer), use a vibrator.

7. Hook your fingers inside you and apply pressure to the front wall of the vagina. Feel for a spongy area about 1 to 1 ½ inches (2.5 to 3.8 cm) inside. Press and rub the area; notice how your body responds. You're looking for an area that's sensitive when you apply firm pressure—the G-spot prefers firm pressure to gentle stroking.

8. Another signal that you've found the right spot is you might feel the urge to pee. The urethral sponge surrounds the urethra, so it makes sense, and it's a very common feeling.

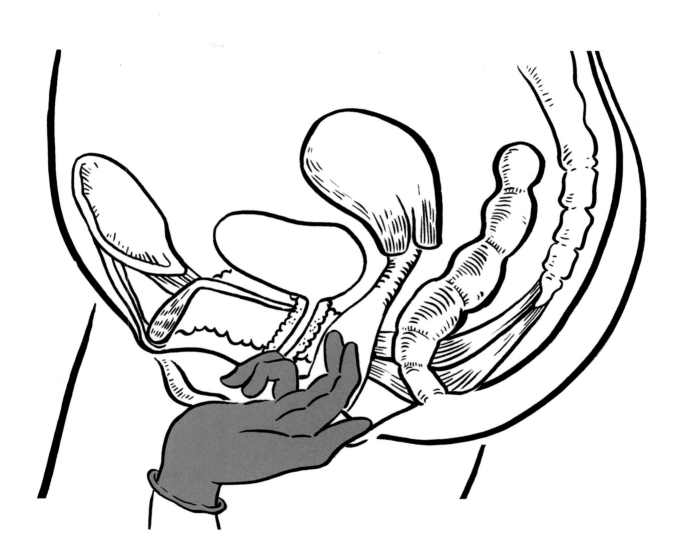

CHAPTER 3

TAKE MATTERS INTO YOUR OWN HANDS: SOLO G-SPOT STIMULATION

G-spot stimulation ups the intensity so much, but it also is a signal to me that I've hit a richer level of arousal. If I'm not ready for it yet, pressing against my G-spot feels unpleasant and annoying. But once I'm turned on enough for it, it offers a very deep, rumbling, emanating, inviting, powerful, erotic connection to my body and my sensuality. I'm aware of my sexual pleasure in a different way, in a way that draws my attention to my own ability to feel that pleasure. It starts at my core and radiates outward, but it's not as though I can feel my toes tingling. Instead, it's as though my whole body is my G-spot. My whole body wants and demands and feels pleasure, and I become open to wrapping myself around that source of pleasure until my whole body is satisfied.

—Rose

Some women find their G-spots for the first time while masturbating, which makes sense. When you want to try something new, it's often easier to do it on your own. After all, who knows your body better than you? You know the hot spots, the buttons to push, and what gets you revved up. You can go at your own pace, try different techniques, change positions, whatever you want. You can be picky, frustrated, giddy, turned on—all on your own terms. Practicing by yourself takes pressure off the situation. Sometimes, when you try something new with a partner, you want it to go well or you want to please him or her, which adds a stressful element. When those kinds of pressures are off the table, you can relax into the experience without worry. Remember, the more you have sex with yourself, the better you'll be at having sex with your partner.

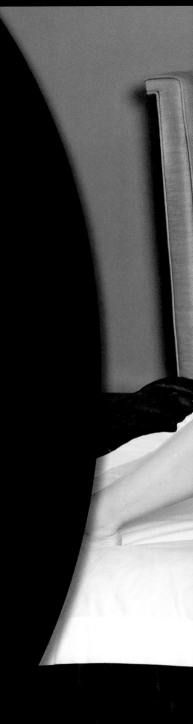

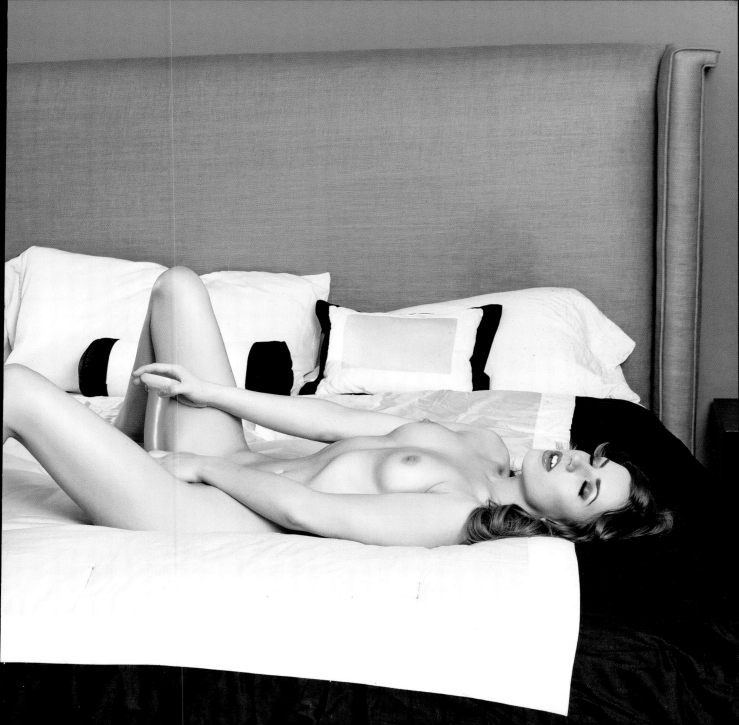

Masturbation can also be about information gathering for partnered sex; you can try out a bunch of things, and then report back to your partner. The more you know about your own body—what you like, what you don't, what feels good, what doesn't, what turns you on, what turns you off—the more you can share these valuable details. It's a win-win situation: You'll feel more comfortable with the new activity, and your partner will be grateful for your discoveries. If you find your G-spot on your own, you can help guide your partner there. If you stumble on a technique that really worked for you, you can share it with him or her. If you try a new toy that floats your boat, you can incorporate it into your lovemaking. And, if you're not too shy, you can masturbate *for* your partner. This is a big turn-on for lots of people, but it's not just about putting on a hot show. When you demonstrate exactly what you like, your partner can take mental notes and use them later to touch you in similar ways.

THE MIND-BODY CONNECTION

The power of positive thinking is real, and it goes a long way when it comes to our sexual explorations. Begin your G-spot exploration with a sense of wonder, curiosity, and enthusiasm; banish self-judgment and silence negative voices. Be open to something new.

- Make sure you're in the right frame of mind before you begin your G-spot adventure.

- Be willing to go wherever the sexual experience takes you.

- Drop your expectations—don't put pressure on yourself, and don't have a goal in mind.

- Don't go into the experience insisting you must enjoy G-spot stimulation and it must make you come. That's just a recipe for disaster.

- Be open to new sensations and different feelings.

Sometimes, you can be mentally ready, but you're not in the same place physically. Your body may need some time to catch up with your brain, and that is okay. If you are not aroused, stimulation and penetration can be uncomfortable (or even painful) because your body isn't ready for intense sensations. Listen to your body and don't try to rush the arousal process. Remember that the more revved up your engine is, the easier it will be to find the G-spot and the better it will feel when you stimulate it.

BEST POSITIONS FOR G-SPOTTING ON YOUR OWN

Lots of women have a favorite masturbation position, and that's definitely the best place to start. When you're ready to explore your G-spot, here are some suggestions for different positions that will give you a good angle to find and stimulate the spot. Many women masturbate on their backs, but there are several ways you can adapt this position to maximize its potential. Experiment with these positions to see which ones work best for you.

1. Lie on your back with a pillow under your butt; the pillow helps tilt your pelvis upward. In this position, whether you're using your fingers or a toy, aim up toward the front of your body. In one variation, if it's comfortable, you bring your knees to your chest. This is like folding your body in half, so it may not be sustainable for people with limited flexibility or mobility. But if it works for you, this position can make it easier for you to reach your G-spot with your fingers.

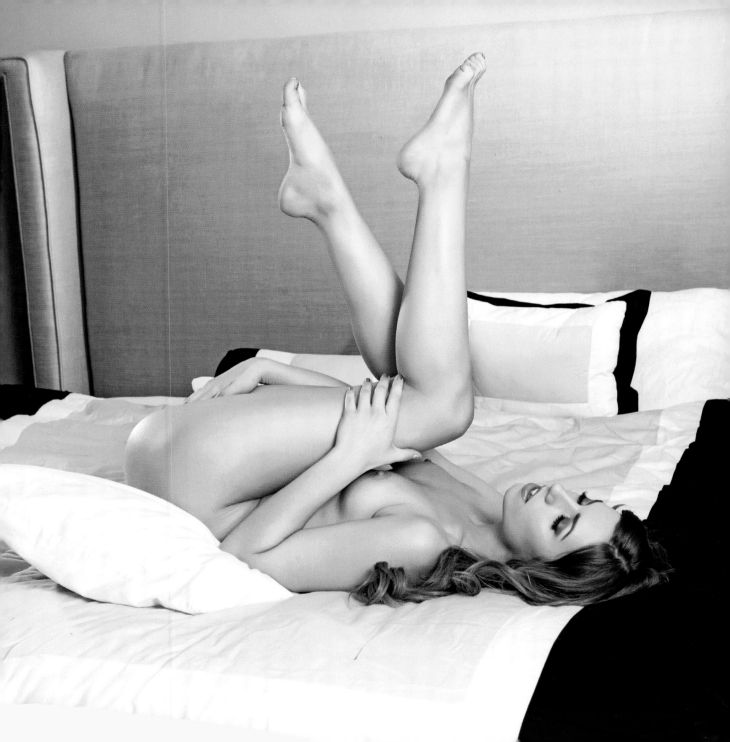

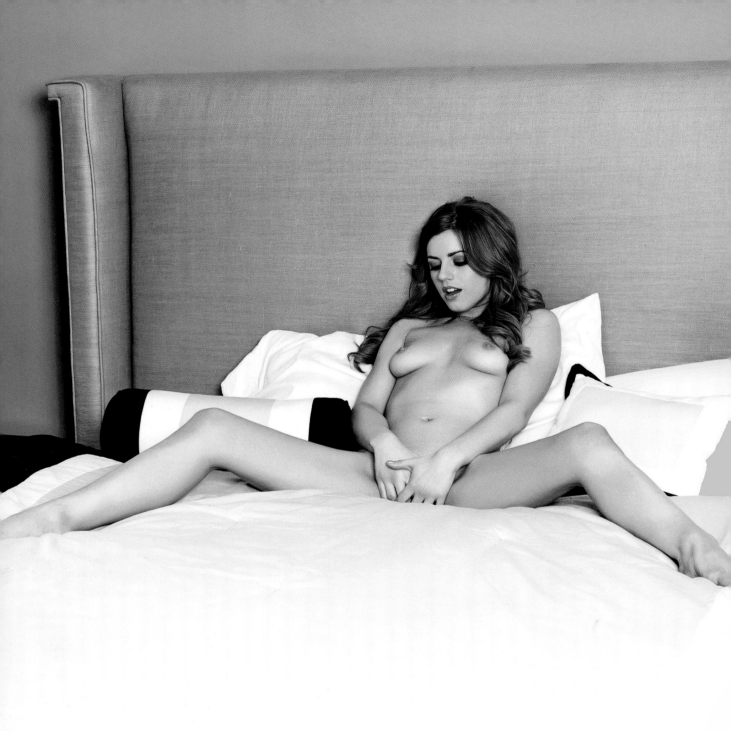

2. Another option is to sit up with your back supported (against the headboard of your bed, for example) and your legs out straight so they form a 90-degree angle to your torso. This is a better position if you have back issues than lying completely flat on your back, and makes it easier to maneuver your hands and/or a toy.

3. Masturbating on your stomach is a much more difficult position for solitary G-spot exploration—it's tricky enough to slide your fingers inside you in that position, let alone curve them to hit the G-spot. A toy is a better choice, although it may still be more difficult to maneuver than if you were lying on your back. A vibrator works best in this position because the vibration alone can stimulate the G-spot. Add some hip motion and rocking.

4. If you like toys and prefer partnered positions where you're on top, try this one. Kneel on the bed and sit back on your calves. Bring the toy between your legs and slide it inside you. Adjust your body by tilting your hips to find the best angle. Aim the toy up and forward so it's pressing against the G-spot.

5. Do you like to masturbate in the shower or bathtub? Try a dildo with a suction cup on the end, and suction it to the bottom of the tub. Straddle the dildo by sitting on your knees or squatting over it. Use your hands on the side of the tub for leverage. This way, you can ride the dildo, controlling the angle and depth of penetration.

SOLO G-SPOT EXPLORATION AND STIMULATION

When you begin masturbating, remind yourself that this is your time. You're not trying to have a quick orgasm to get off, relieve stress, or help you fall asleep. Settle in for a longer-than-usual session. Spend some time exploring your body, keeping in mind that the more time you give yourself, the easier it will be to find your G-spot.

1. Start by massaging the inner and outer labia, using some lube or wetness from your vagina.

2. Tease the vaginal opening and notice how your body responds to your touch.

3. When you're ready, begin to play with your clitoris. You may like long, slow strokes at first, pressure on the hood above the clitoral shaft, or a circular motion with two fingers. You know your body best; you know what gets you going. Take your time and let the arousal build.

4. As you feel your body relax and you get increasingly turned on, work your way up to penetration. Bring your hand in front of you between your legs and bend your elbow and wrist so that your palm faces you with your fingers down.

5. Slide your middle finger inside your vagina and start to slowly slide it in and out. Add another finger if you want.

6. Hook your fingers and press against the front wall with your fingertips as you feel for your G-spot, that spongy area about 1 to 1½ inches (2.5 to 3.8 cm) inside.

7. Remember, you are stimulating the urethral sponge through the front wall of the vagina—it's not right there at your fingertips, so to speak. That's why the G-spot prefers firm pressure to gentle stroking.

8. You might feel the urge to pee. When you stimulate the sponge, the urethra is also stimulated, sending a signal to your brain that you have to pee. You may have felt a similar sensation during masturbation or sex with a partner. Some women actually enjoy the sensation, which doesn't feel at all like they're stuck in traffic miles from the nearest rest stop. Instead, it feels quite pleasurable. For some women, it may feel strange; just like anything new, it takes some getting used to. The important thing is not to panic—panic is counterproductive to pleasure. If it's simply too distracting or annoying to you, back off on the stimulation and try again another time.

9. If you get over the pee feeling, experiment with different stimulation techniques to see what feels good to you. Take long strokes, and then short ones. Use one finger, and then see how it feels when you insert more. Try the "come here" technique—curve your fingers and make a pulling motion away from you. The hand position and motion may sound awkward. That's because it is. In truth, it's difficult for some women to find their G-spots with their own fingers— they just can't contort their bodies to make it work. It can be frustrating, so don't worry if it's not working for you on your own. All hope is not lost. Other women can find their G-spots, but may not be able to stimulate it with enough intensity for it to be pleasurable. That's where a good G-spot toy enters the picture.

10. G-spot toys make finding the G-spot ergonomically easier and less awkward than using your fingers. Toys can provide the vigorous stimulation the G-spot likes, but that you can't achieve with your own hand. A toy can stimulate the clitoris when you've run out of hands or can't reach it when your fingers are otherwise engaged. Toys designed to make the G-spot sing should be part of your toolbox.

GOOD VIBRATIONS: MY FAVORITE TOYS FOR SOLO PLAY

These are my picks for some of the best of the best. I chose them because they are easy to handle on your own; however, all these toys can be used with a partner as well.

SUPER SOLO DILDO: G-FORCE

When choosing a dildo for yourself, make sure it's long enough to easily hold and maneuver; I suggest a minimum of 6 inches (15 cm). The silicone dildo called G-Force, made by Tantus, is longer than most dildos (more than 10 inches [25 cm]) and you can get a good grip on the textured handle at the end. Having a good grip is important when lube drips down your hand and things get slippery! It's not an anatomically realistic-looking dildo, but it does have a nice teardrop-shaped head that makes it great for G-spot stimulation. It's flexible enough to curve toward the G-spot, but firm enough to provide excellent stimulation.

WAND FOR ONE: THE WAVE

Individually handmade of more than 8 inches (20 cm) of clear borosilicate glass, The Wave from PyreXions is amazing. One end has a smooth, curved shaft with a bulbous head, and the other has multiple beads. Insert the smoother end into your vagina, and the curve lines right up with the G-spot. Hold on to the beaded end and get ready for some fantastic sensations. Use a press-and-pull motion with this toy—press the head against your G-spot, then pull the toy out less than 1 inch (2.5 cm); you're basically twisting your wrist. The solid glass surface will press firmly against your G-spot.

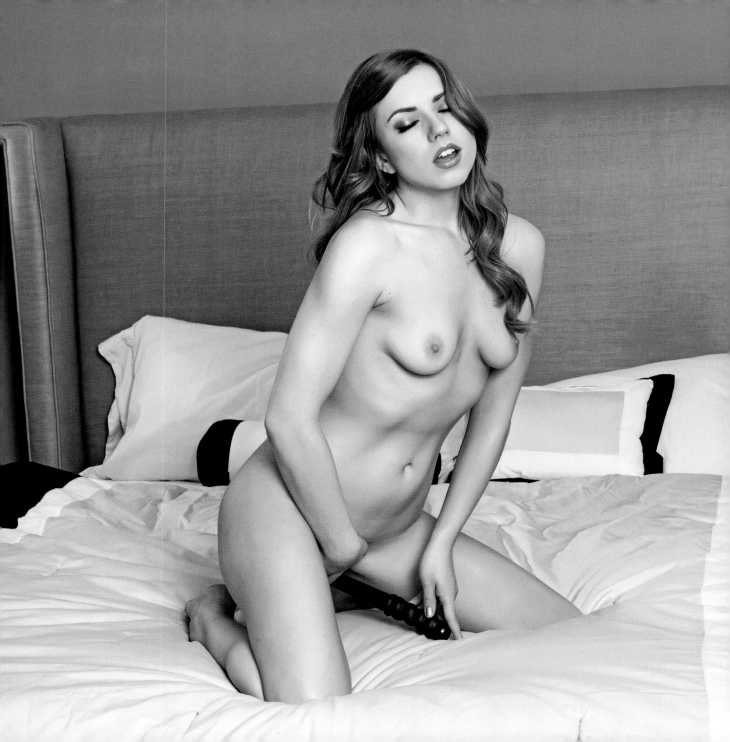

PERMISSION FOR PLEASURE

Erotic touch is a gift, but it's one we don't give ourselves often enough. For many people, the first sexual partners we have are ourselves, and masturbation is the way we are introduced to sex. It is important to make time for masturbation, whether you have sexual partners or not. It's an opportunity to connect with your body, tap into your sexuality, develop and explore fantasies, and try new things. Self-knowledge is the key to sexual health, well-being, and pleasure. It's something women often don't make time for: a space that is all about *you*.

Making an erotic date with yourself may feel strange at first, but it's an important part of maintaining your connection to your sexual self. Create a time and space that are judgment-free, where you give yourself permission to try anything without goals or expectations. When you forge and nurture a sexual self-connection, you can work on letting go of any shame and embarrassment you might have, become more comfortable with your body, and increase your sexual confidence.

VIRTUOUS VIBRATOR: GIGI

The Swedish company Lelo makes high-quality, super-quiet, gorgeously designed and packaged vibrators (and other toys). Whereas most vibes have a smooth tapered end or a bulbous head, Lelo's GIGI has a firm raised end with a nearly flat surface. This provides more surface area to press against the G-spot. GIGI is made of medical-grade silicone and hard plastic and is rechargeable (it stays charged for about an hour). But what sets it apart from other vibrators is its unique shape and design. The GIGI is 6½ inches (16.5 cm) long (with 4½ inches [11.5 cm] making up the insertable portion) and has a very subtle curve. It's especially good for women who've found that other insertable vibrators are too long or the curve is too drastic and doesn't work for them. You can adjust the speed to your taste and choose from five different vibration modes: a constant vibration, three pulsing vibrations (slow, medium, and fast intervals), and "before and after" mode during which the vibration builds to a strong surge, then backs off, then builds again. If you're looking for more length and girth, try Lelo's Mona vibrator.

⌕ TRISTAN'S TIPS
Here's a tip to try with the GIGI (and other insertable vibrators). Slide it inside, angle it so it presses against the front wall of the vagina, and let it vibrate against the G-spot. Rather than moving it in and out, see what vibration and pressure alone feel like. For some women, it's not about thrusting motion.

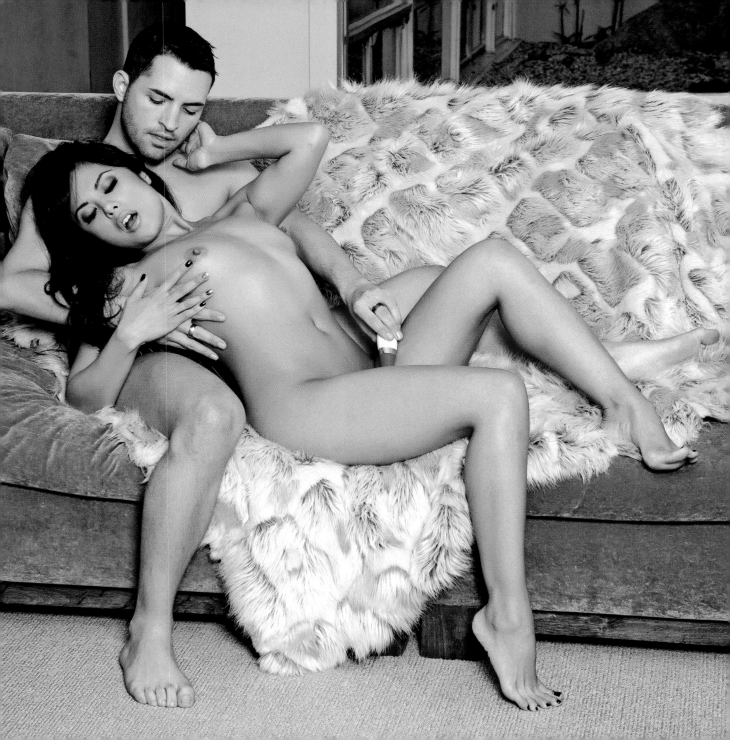

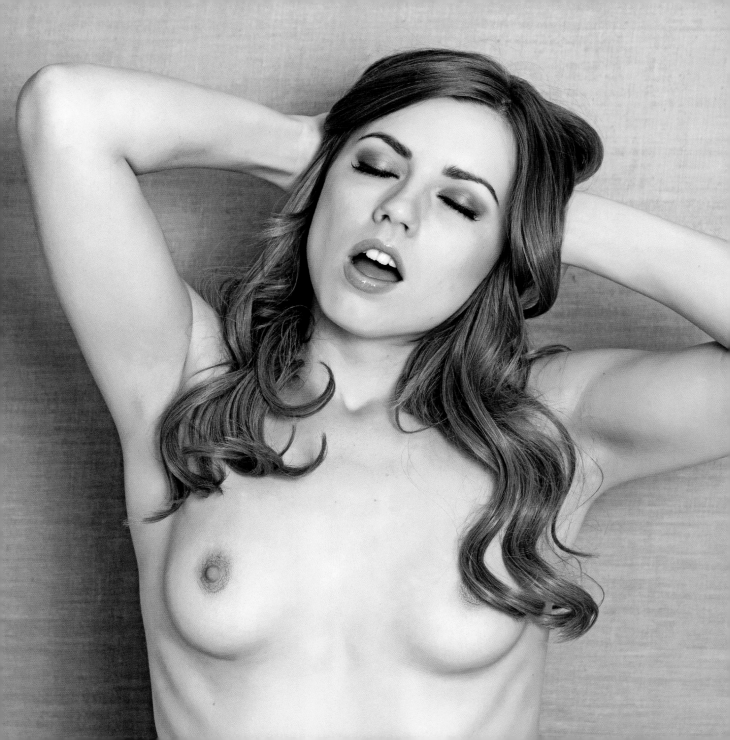

DELIGHTFUL DUAL-ACTION: ROCK CHICK

Are you someone who needs clitoral stimulation with any kind of penetration? Or do you find that without clit stimulation, working your G-spot doesn't feel as pleasurable? Then try a dual-action vibrator for simultaneous clitoral and G-spot stimulation. The Rock Chick is a silicone U-shaped, battery-powered vibrator made by the British company Rocks Off Ltd. The smooth part of the Rock Chick goes inside your vagina, and its exaggerated curve targets the sensitive G-spot, while the ridged end hugs your clitoris and vulva. It's got a unique ergonomic shape that's different from most vibrators—it can be easier to use on yourself because the external part is right within reach.

Rather than using the toy like a dildo or an insertable vibe with a straight in-and-out motion, you make a much shallower rocking motion with the Rock Chick. You can hold on to the ridged part and press the toy inside you. You can grip the middle of the U like a handle and move the toy that way. Or you can use it hands-free and let the vibration do all the work. The Rock Chick is designed to stimulate the G-spot and the clitoris at the same time, but remember that every woman's body is different; everything may not "line up" in exactly the places you need it to be. Because the Rock Chick is flexible, you can experiment with different placements. Or, with the toy inside you, try rocking your hips upward to meet the outer part with your clitoris.

AMAZING ATTACHMENT: GEE WHIZ

The Hitachi Magic Wand is one of the most popular clitoral vibrators on the market and has been for years. The Magic Wand has a body the size of a paper towel roll (just the cardboard roll, without the paper towels) and a flexible, cushiony plastic head the size of a tennis ball and the shape of a marshmallow. Because it plugs in, it offers more power than battery-operated and rechargeable vibrators, and in it is considered the most powerful vibrator on the market.

You can transform your Hitachi Magic Wand into a G-spot toy with Gee Whiz, the ingenious silicone attachment made by Vixen Creations. The Gee Whiz fits over the head of the Magic Wand and converts into an insertable vibrator. Because the attachment is silicone, it conducts that powerful vibration beautifully and evenly throughout. Plus, once you slide the attachment inside you, the head of the Magic Wand sits against your vulva and hugs your clit.

Now you're ready to build your very own toolbox for G-spot adventures. Read the next chapter to find out about different toys designed especially to entice the G-spot and learn how to pick the right lubricants for you.

CHAPTER 4

YOUR G-SPOT TOOLBOX

Measly words can't adequately describe what the Pure Wand feels like. This is the most intense, overwhelming sex toy I've ever used. It is heavy, concentrated, and unrelenting. It steals my breath. It messes with my sanity. It says, *HELLO G-SPOT, OH HI THERE, OH HEY*, and it does not stop until I run out of energy and collapse. It gives me goose bumps. It makes me cry. And it leaves me with a puddle of ejaculate underneath me, which then runs down my legs when I stand up.

—Epiphora[8]

As you begin your journey to discovering the pleasures of the G-spot, you'll want to assemble some specific tools to assist you along the way. I've mentioned the importance of lube when it comes to penetration, and here we dig into the details of all the different kinds. I gave you my picks for some of the best G-spot toys in the previous chapter; the following guide to toys will help you select the right ones for you.

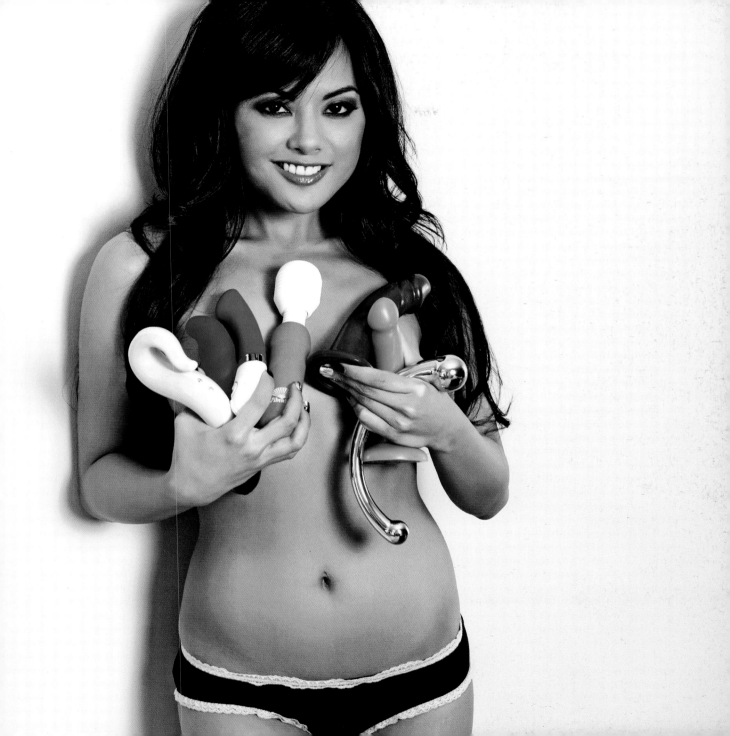

GET READY, GET SET, GET WET!

Because exploring the G-spot involves penetration, you want your vagina to be prepared. As I discussed earlier, during the arousal process, the vaginal walls secrete lubrication. However, the amount of lubrication the vagina produces varies a great deal. Some women get very wet, others get a little wet, and for some, the amount they lubricate can change.

So many different factors can negatively affect the body's ability to lubricate, including your diet, exercise, stress, dehydration, too much coffee or alcohol, and smoking cigarettes or marijuana. When your hormone levels change, you can also experience a decrease in lubrication. Thus your menstrual cycle, pregnancy, childbirth, nursing, perimenopause, menopause, or a hormonal imbalance (including hypothyroidism) can all be factors in how much you lubricate.

Certain products marketed for "feminine hygiene," including douches, scented tampons, feminine sprays, and even harsh soaps, can dry out the delicate tissue and decrease lubrication. Vaginal dryness can be the result of over-the-counter drugs, such as allergy medication, and prescription drugs, including some types of birth control, antibiotics, antidepressants, and sedatives. Some treatments for vaginosis, urinary tract infections (UTIs), ulcers, and high blood pressure can also cause decreased lubrication. In addition, serious illness and its treatment, including cancer and chemotherapy, can result in problems with vaginal lubrication.

LUBE IS YOUR FRIEND

Women and men can feel shy, ambivalent, or even ashamed about using lube, and their feelings are often based on myths and misinformation. Stereotypes may contribute to your attitudes about lube: "If you're turned on, your body should be wet." "Only menopausal women need lube." "If you need lube, something is wrong with you." You have to let go of these ideas because they simply are not true. You have a tool at your disposal that can enhance all kinds of sex. Wetter is better!

It's important to know that you can feel totally turned on, yet your vagina may not produce lubrication. Sometimes, your body just needs a little more time to catch up with your head. Maybe your vagina does lube up, but not necessarily enough to make sexual play comfortable or to make intercourse sustainable for more than a few minutes.

The ass does not produce its own lubrication, so for anal play lubrication is an absolute necessity. Even when your play does not include vaginal or anal penetration, the idea of dry skin on skin or a dry toy against the delicate, sensitive skin of the genitals just isn't as appealing as one with a dab of lube to smooth out any friction against the skin. The bottom line is you need lube.

As a general rule, lube should feel good on and in your genitals. If you experience itching, burning, redness, or any kind of irritation, you likely have a sensitivity or an allergy to one or more ingredients in the lube. Everyone's body responds differently to every lube. Don't be discouraged if your first lube adventure ends in a warm shower to rinse it off because it didn't feel good. You simply haven't found the right lube for you. You'll know when you do because it will feel warm, wet, and comfortable. The right lube is a very personal choice. Your best bet is to go to a reputable sex shop or website and get sample sizes of several different brands and try them out. You may end up with a few you like, or one for external stimulation and vaginal intercourse and another for anal play. Read labels carefully; if you're not sure what's in a lube, ask the retailer or manufacturer.

WATER-BASED LUBES

The majority of lubricants on the market are water-based. Water-based lubes are non-staining, are easy to clean up, and come in a variety of brands with different ingredients, consistencies, and tastes. They are compatible with all sex toy materials as well as safer-sex barriers such as latex and non-latex condoms.

Water-based lubes cover the spectrum in terms of consistency: They can be thin and liquidy, medium thickness, or super thick like hair gel. Thin, slippery lubes are meant to mimic vaginal fluids, and work well for vaginal penetration, whereas thicker lubes tend to stay wet longer and work better for anal penetration. The most common complaint about this kind of lube is that it tends to become sticky, stringy, or tacky as time goes by; it also dries up, because it gets absorbed into genital tissue. So, you need to re-lubricate—by adding saliva, water, or more lube—several times, which for some people breaks up the momentum of sex.

⌇ TRISTAN'S TIPS
Popular brands of lube include Astroglide, Durex, K-Y, ID Glide, Pink Water, Probe, Swiss Navy H2O, System JO H2O, and Wet.

Keep in mind that if you plan on putting your mouth where your hands, toys, or a penis has been, you should select a lube with a taste you find palatable. Some water-based lubes, for example, have a bitter or chemical taste that really turns people off. If taste is a big issue for you, choose a flavored lube.

Mmm . . . Tasty: Flavored Water-Based Lubes

Are you someone who doesn't stick to one sexual activity for a very long time? Do you like to switch things up frequently, moving from fingers, to oral, to toys, a little more oral, add some more fingers, and . . . you get the idea. The last thing your lover wants to see is your head pop up from between his or her legs with an awful look on your face. If your mouth is frequently in the mix and you're using plenty of lube, you may want to consider a flavored lube because you're going to be tasting it often.

⌇ TRISTAN'S TIPS
Many of the major brands of lube offer a flavored variety (or varieties), including Astroglide, ID, O'My, Sliquid, Swiss Navy, System JO, and Wet.

Extra Sensitive: Natural, Glycerin-Free, and Organic Lubes

Just as more and more people are buying natural food and beauty products without harmful chemical ingredients, many consumers want their lube to be as natural as possible or organic. Natural and organic lubes are glycerin-, paraben-, and chemical-free, and contain botanicals and plant extracts such as aloe vera. Some come in earth-friendly packaging.

⌇ TRISTAN'S TIPS
Popular brands include Hathor Aphrodisia, Sliquid Organics, Sensua Organics, Intimate Organics, Blossom Organics, and Good Clean Love (which contains organic vegetable glycerin that does not encourage yeast growth as synthetic glycerin does).

G-SPOT GELS AND CREAMS: FRIEND OR FOE?

In recent years, creams and gels to help you find your G-spot have emerged with names such as Ooh! That's It! G-Spot Gel or G-Spot Cream. These lubes help cause the G-spot to swell, thus making it easier to find. The active ingredient in most of these gels is L-arginine (which purportedly increases circulation), menthol or peppermint oil (which creates a tingling/cooling sensation), or both.

Some of these ingredients can irritate some people's genital tissue, so be careful. Plenty of women buy these products, and some really like them. These lubes do create a tingling sensation of some kind inside the vagina, but they won't necessarily help you find your G-spot or intensify its stimulation. You are welcome to try them, but the techniques in this book are more likely to help than any specific product.

Until fairly recently, most water-based lubricants contained glycerin, a common ingredient that helps lube retain its consistency. However, glycerin is a kind of sugar, and yeast feeds on sugar, so many women find that these lubes can cause a vaginal yeast imbalance or a yeast infection. If you are especially prone to yeast infections, or you find that after having sex with a water-based lube you begin to develop symptoms, you should consider a glycerin-free lube. Although glycerin is still on the ingredient list of many water-based lubes, luckily, manufacturers have responded to women's needs for an alternative.

⟁ TRISTAN'S TIPS

You'll find a growing number of glycerin-free lubes on the market, including Frolic, Gun Oil H2O, Hydra-Smooth, Liquid Silk, Maximus, Slippery Stuff, and Sliquid.

In addition to concerns about glycerin, the safety of parabens has been questioned recently. Parabens are petroleum-based chemicals that discourage the growth of bacteria. They are commonly used as preservatives in cosmetics, beauty products, and lubricants. Some studies have linked parabens to weight gain, skin problems, and certain types of cancer. If you are concerned about parabens, read labels carefully (benzyl, butyl, ethyl, isobutyl, methyl, and propyl are all parabens).

⟁ TRISTAN'S TIPS

Several lubricant makers offer glycerin-free and paraben-free varieties, including Astroglide Glycerin/Paraben Free, ID Moments, Ride, Sliquid (all varieties), and Wet Naturals for Women.

Stoke the Fires: Warming Lubes

One trend in the water-based lube marketplace is lube that creates a warming sensation on contact, and nearly all the major brands have produced one. When you apply these lubes to your genitals, they create a warming sensation that sends blood rushing to the area, which helps the arousal process. The main ingredient differs: It might be acacia honey or a derivative (found in Astroglide Warming Liquid, Wet Warming Lubricant, and K-Y Warming Liquid); menthol (in ID Sensation, Hot Elbow Grease, and the glycerin-free Sliquid Sizzle); or, the most natural of them all, cinnamon bark (in Emerita OH).

As with lube in general, whether you like it is totally a matter of personal preference. Some people find the sensation to be subtle and they love how it makes their private parts tingle. Some women find it helps them get turned on faster. Others say the feeling is similar to sticking Bengay in your vagina or butt—it's way too intense and feels more annoying than pleasurable.

SILICONE LUBES

Silicone lubes are non-staining and often flavorless. They are more expensive than water-based ones, but you use a lot less because they don't dry up as easily. They tend to be super-concentrated and a little bit goes a long way. Many people prefer the slick texture of silicone and the fact that many of these lubes don't get sticky or tacky as some water-based lubes can.

Silicone lubes work with condoms and other safer-sex barriers as well as some sex toy materials, including PVC, rubber, glass, hard plastic, acrylic, and metal. However, silicone lubes are *not* compatible with CyberSkin or silicone sex toys and will ruin them (cover these toys with condoms to protect them or use a different kind of lube). Silicone lube is perfect for sex in a shower or bath because it stays slick underwater, whereas water-based lubes don't.

⌕ TRISTAN'S TIPS
Lubricants made with silicone are gaining popularity and include such brands as Eros, Eros Gel, Astroglide X, Swiss Navy Silicone, System JO Original, Sliquid Silver, Gun Oil, Wet Platinum, K-Y Intrigue, and ID Velvet.

LUBES TO AVOID

Oil-Based Lubes

Most oil-based lubes on the market contain mineral oil, coconut oil, almond oil, vegetable oil, or some combination; they work well for male masturbation and hand jobs. Many of them are formulated with ingredients that won't stain fabrics, but read the label carefully because they can be hard to clean up.

Oil-based lubes can break down latex condoms and many toy materials, but their biggest danger is to vaginas. If any oil lube gets inside one, you can't rinse or douche it out. It will linger in a vagina, providing an ideal environment for bacteria to grow, causing a vaginal infection. If you are going to use them for a hand job during partnered sex and you want to have intercourse or any kind of penetration afterward, be sure to wash the lube off his hands, your hands, and his penis, then switch to another kind of lube.

Novelty Creams and Lubes

A holdover from the old days of "adult novelties," some lubes promise things like "Stay Harder Longer," "More Enjoyable Anal Sex," or "Tighten Your Vagina for a Better Orgasm" right on the package. Beware! Lubes with names such as Magic Stamina or Anal Eze contain benzocaine or another topical anesthetic. They numb whatever they touch: a penis, a vagina, an anus. When you use them, you're more likely to go farther or take something bigger than you're ready for. So-called "vaginal tightening" lubes contain either benzocaine (to numb tissue and reduce lubrication) or a tissue-shrinking astringent (such as aleppo oak gall or potassium alum); not only are they a marketing gimmick that reeks of sexism, but they also don't really work and can irritate vaginal tissue.

HYBRID LUBES: THE BEST OF BOTH WORLDS

Liquid Silk, Sliquid Silk Hybrid Formula, and Gun Oil Force Recon are water-silicone hybrid lubes. They combine the easy-to-clean, non-staining properties of a glycerin-free, water-based lube with the staying power of a silicone lube. Liquid Silk is safe to use with most silicone toys. Sliquid Silk Hybrid Formula is 12 percent silicone and doesn't contain parabens. Although the manufacturers play it safe and recommend you don't use them with silicone toys, some people say it's safe with the best-quality silicone (including Vixen and Tantus).

G-SPOT TOYS: YOUR PATH TO SOLO AND PARTNERED PLEASURE

Plenty of myths exist about sex toys: "Toys are for people who can't get 'the real thing.'" "If you need a toy, something must be wrong with you or your partner must lack skills." "Good lovers don't need any help from a toy." Let's clear up these misguided beliefs and expose the truth.

Spinsters, antisocial loners, and the sexually dysfunctional aren't keeping sex toy companies in business—people from all walks of life, both single and partnered, regularly use sex toys. Sex toys are not replacements for partners, and people don't always use them *instead* of having partnered sex. If a person feels threatened by sex toys, he may believe that his partner's desire for a toy is a not-so-subtle comment on his skill as a lover. Using a toy is not about compensating for your shortcomings, however; it's about bringing something new into the mix to enhance sex. Some toys do things human beings simply can't, such as deliver powerful, consistent clitoral stimulation.

Sex toys are designed for pleasure, and they can benefit your sex life in many different ways. In addition to boosting the arousal process, expanding your sexual repertoire, delivering unique kinds of stimulation, and helping bring you to orgasm, they are great for G-spot exploration. Using a toy while you masturbate is a good way to find your own G-spot, learn more about your body, experiment with different kinds of stimulation, and see what really works for you. With a partner, sex toys can help you move away from an intercourse-always model of sex.

Intercourse is often seen as the ultimate activity, the one you're working your way toward—the main event. But the truth is that intercourse isn't the only way to have sex. It's not the best way to locate the G-spot, and for many women, it's not always the best way to stimulate the G-spot. Sex toys can also give you an "extra set of hands" in the bedroom, allowing you to do two or more things at once. Imagine being able to focus all your attention on giving amazing oral sex while an insertable vibrator works her G-spot. Or you could focus on putting the exact pressure she likes on her G-spot while a vibrator stimulates her clitoris. The possibilities are endless!

You'll find a huge selection of sex toys on the market, and choosing one can be a challenge, especially for beginners. I suggest that you go to a local, female-friendly store where toys are displayed out of their packaging. This way, you see a toy's exact size, feel its material and texture, turn it on, hear how much noise it makes, feel how powerful the vibration is, and determine how easy it is to use. Plus, you can ask a staffer for tips, advice, and recommendations. An in-person purchase can make all the difference in getting exactly what you want.

If that's not possible, then pick a reputable website from which to make your purchase. Look for these elements: detailed product descriptions written by the staff, unbiased customer reviews, and customer service by phone. Here are some of the different categories of G-spot toys available.

HOMING IN ON THE G-SPOT WITH DILDOS

Dildos are non-vibrating insertable toys designed for penetration. Plenty of couples use dildos for all kinds of sex play, and they are especially helpful for G-spot stimulation. Why? Because you can choose the exact length, width, and curve of a dildo—the perfect one for you. You can't do that with a penis. And, if your male partner comes before you do, a dildo keeps the penetration going.

Realistic and semi-realistic dildos with circumcised heads make great G-spot toys, because the head is a perfect stimulator. You'll also find less realistic dildos that have a pronounced curve designed especially for stimulating the G-spot.

Dildos come in a variety of materials, but most are made of rubber, softened PVC, vinyl, thermoplastic rubber (TPR), or silicone. They vary in length and width, and can be as modest as the size of a finger or as grand as a tall soda can. Some dildos resemble penises; others are simply phallic in shape. Most dildos are made to be compatible with dildo harnesses, so with a partner you can strap them on if you wish.

Partners of either gender can feel threatened or uneasy with dildo play, and some men in particular may have a hard time with it. If your male partner feels this way, remind him that you want *him* to use the dildo on you, and without him, it won't be as much fun. Help him realize that a dildo isn't a cop-out, and sex does not always have to revolve around his penis. Guys, remember a dildo may not be part of your body, but when it's in your hand, you're the one who's going to get the credit for showing your girl a great time. And take it from me: She will have a great time.

Flexible Dildos

If you're looking for a flexible dildo, I always recommend silicone (such as the G-Force dildo I described in the previous chapter). Silicone is durable and easy to clean. It can be disinfected, warms to body temperature, and conducts vibration best. Because silicone is not porous like other soft materials, silicone toys can be disinfected and shared by different partners. Silicone is the most expensive of the soft materials, but it's worth it. It is very resilient, so it will last through years of use. The only drawback is that you cannot use silicone lubricants with toys made of silicone; most silicone lube bonds to a silicone toy and ruins it, so stick to water-based lubes.

⌕ TRISTAN'S TIPS
Make sure you purchase toys made of medical-grade or platinum silicone. You can contact toy manufacturers and inquire about what kind of silicone they use in their toys, or buy toys made by companies with a reputation for top-quality silicone, such as Vixen Creations (which offers a lifetime warranty on its toys), Fun Factory, Tantus Silicone, and Jollies.

If you're looking for something less expensive, you can choose a dildo made of rubber, vinyl, thermal plastic, or softened PVC (polyvinyl chloride, plus softening agents known as phthalates). These toys are cheap to produce and thus more affordable. They come in a wide variety of styles, from super-realistic flesh-toned to colorful and glittery. These toys are not long-term investments; they definitely have a shelf life and should be replaced regularly (at least once a year).

Because they are porous, you should never share these toys unless you cover them with condoms. Recently, there has been some serious debate about the safety of softened PVC toys, because they contain chemicals known as phthalates (which some people believe to be unsafe and potentially toxic). If you want to know if a soft toy contains phthalates, ask the company or look for telltale signs: a distinct plastic odor and a greasy film. Some companies have developed soft plastics without these chemicals, so if this is a concern for you, look for toys made of elastomer or those marked "phthalate-free."

Strap-on Harnesses for Dildos

Strap-ons are a great way to experience hands-free penetrative sex for women who have sex with women, as well as for men with erectile dysfunction or those who want to last all night long. Strap-on sex can also be part of fantasy role-playing or gender play for some people. It's a chance for couples to incorporate a sex toy into their bedroom routine in a new way.

Some strap-on dildos and harnesses are sold together in kits, but the best strap-on is the one you build yourself by choosing the dildo and the harness separately. Harnesses can be made of leather, vinyl, nylon, rubber, and other kinds of fabric. They have three different types of fasteners: metal D-rings, through which the material slides; plastic fasteners similar to straps on a backpack; or metal buckles like those on a belt. Harnesses come in a variety of styles and can be basic, embellished, no-nonsense, or glamorous. You can embrace a fetish look with leather and metal hardware, go for a superhero image with a red sparkly harness, or even choose a clear plastic see-through harness.

In addition to aesthetics, harnesses come in two main styles: one-strap and two-strap. A one-strap harness has a strap that goes around your hips, a strap that goes between your legs, and a panel in front (sometimes with a cock ring) where the dildo slips through a hole. Because it fits like a G-string, the center strap rubs against your genitals, which may feel stimulating to some people and annoying to others. This style harness tends to fit petite women the best.

A two-strap harness has a strap that goes around your hips and two straps that go around your ass cheeks. It fits like a jockstrap, leaving your vagina and ass easily accessible and free to be stimulated. It has a panel of material in front with a hole for the dildo and a cock ring. Some two-strap models have just a cock ring without a panel of material. Some styles have a detachable cock ring that can be changed to accommodate different size dildos. These are especially good if the dildo you are using is significantly smaller or larger than average. Others have a cock ring that sits on top of the material, so the base of the dildo does not fit directly against your body. Some people find that the two-strap harness gives them more control than the one-strap model because the dildo moves around less and is easier to guide.

Choose a harness that fits you well—the snugger and more secure the better. If you are a larger woman, ask the store for harnesses designed for large women or whether you can order extra-long straps. I recommend that you try on a few different styles before you buy one; most reputable stores will let you try it on over your clothes. If you order from a catalog or website, check out the return policy. The majority of dildos will fit in a standard harness, as long as there is a flared base and the dildo isn't excessively large.

Remember, if you're using a very curved dildo the curve should always be aimed toward the front of the woman's body. For example, if your partner moves from being on her back to being on all fours, you may want to move the dildo in the harness 180 degrees so that the curve is headed for the G-spot. Plenty of people don't change the dildo's direction and still get great G-spot stimulation with certain angles and positions.

STIMULATING WORKS OF ART: WANDS

Some people consider all insertable toys dildos, but I make a distinction between dildos and wands. Wands are insertable non-vibrating toys designed for handheld use—they can't be worn in a strap-on harness. Wands tend to be less phallic, and are more likely to come in creative shapes and be curved like a U or an S, or some variation. They are most often made of solid or firm materials such as glass, metal, wood, or hard plastic. Both their curved shape and their hard texture make wands ideal toys for G-spot stimulation. The G-spot responds to firm, deliberate pressure, so many people find a toy with a solid surface works much better than one made of a pliable material. Because of their high-quality materials, wands tend to be expensive, and many cost more than $100.

Glass wands are as gorgeous as they are functional. With unique shapes, dazzling colors, and handmade quality, glass wands have become very popular in recent years. They can be fashioned to look like a glass penis, a baton, a curved wand, and even a candy cane! One of the best things about glass is its incredible surface. Even the best-quality silicone toy will have some "drag" to it when you run your fingers along it, but not glass. Glass is seamless and compatible with all kinds of lubricants. People also like glass because it has some weight to it.

⬚ TRISTAN'S TIPS
When you're buying a glass toy, make sure it's made of medical-grade borosilicate, which can withstand extreme heat and cold as well as pressure or shock. Pyrex is one of the most well-known brand names of this type of glass.

Like glass, metal wands are striking in their modern, stream-lined designs. The Pure Wand Epiphora raved about in the opening of this chapter is an example of a stainless steel wand. Wands are smooth and shiny and are often heavier than glass wands. If you like a smooth, firm, solid toy, you'll find a variety of styles as well as weights. Easy to clean and compatible with all lubes, these are some of the best G-spot toys in the world. They're durable and nonporous and conduct hot and cold temperatures nicely. A variety of metal toys are on the market, made of aluminum or stainless steel, some hollow and some of solid metal. Like glass, these toys create an amazingly smooth sensation for penetration and they hold on to lube well.

For people who want a firm, inflexible wand without the price tag of glass or metal, hard plastic is a good alternative. However, some hard plastic toys can be expensive, especially if they are made of medical-grade, nontoxic plastic. Other wands are made of clear acrylic or Lucite (which is a brand name of acrylic). Well-made acrylic toys should be seamless (seams reflect lower quality toys that are mass-produced).

⬚ TRISTAN'S TIPS
Another option, believe it or not, is wood. A boutique company called NobEssence makes sculptural, ergonomic wands (dildos and cock rings, too) of exotic hardwoods, including cocobolo, bamboo, bloodwood, and macassar ebony—all organic and sustainably farmed for those of you who worry about depleting our forests. The toys are hypoallergenic and sealed in a sixteen-step finishing process with Lubrosity (a trade-secret coating), making them waterproof, safe for penetration, and easy to clean.

ADD SOME BUZZ: INSERTABLE VIBRATORS

Insertable vibrators are vibrators designed especially for penetration (rather than external clitoral stimulation). They range in length, from as short as 4 inches (10 cm) to as long as 14 inches (35.5 cm), but most tend to be about 7 to 8 inches (17.5 to 20 cm). These vibrators have a range of girths as well and come in a variety of materials, textures, and styles. They are either battery-powered or rechargeable. Most are phallic-shaped or curved (with shapes similar to wands), rather than being designed to look like penises, but their aesthetics vary a great deal.

Many insertable vibrators are designed specifically for G-spot stimulation, and you can tell because they have a distinctive curve (as opposed to a straight phallic shape). Some have bulbous heads, have balls on the end, or resemble a crooked finger. The end of the toy is designed to aim directly for that sensitive spot on the front wall of the vagina. Most vibrators in this style are made of hard plastic, softer PVC, elastomer, silicone, or some combination.

Vibration is a great way to "wake up" the G-spot. Sometimes, you can slide a vibrator inside and let it just vibrate against the front wall—no in-and-out thrusting, just keep it still. The fast and powerful pulsing of a vibrator increases circulation and gets the blood pumping to the urethral sponge. As more blood rushes to the area, the sponge starts to swell and becomes more prominent and more sensitive. Once the sponge becomes swollen, you can begin moving the toy inside you; the vibration will continue to feel amazing, massaging the urethral sponge through the front wall. The vibration creates a rippling effect that resonates throughout the entire genital area. For some women, the combination of firm pressure and vibration is exactly what their G-spots respond to. In other words, dildos and wands feel great, but toys that vibrate add another dimension.

TWICE THE FUN: DUAL-ACTION VIBRATORS

Dual-action vibrators are the ultimate multitasking sex toys: They deliver penetration and clitoral stimulation simultaneously. The clitoris is a key erogenous zone for the majority of women, and many need some kind of clitoral stimulation during sex play. It helps turn them on and keep them that way—the clit always has to be in the mix. For some, clitoral stimulation heightens the pleasure of penetration and of G-spot stimulation. If that describes you, then a dual-action G-spot toy is your best choice. These toys come in two basic types with some variation: rabbit style and curved double action.

Rabbit-Style Vibes

Rabbit-style vibrators are probably the best known and most recognizable. I call this kind of toy "rabbit style" because most people know the Rabbit Pearl, made famous by Samantha in *Sex and the City*. The design of these toys is pretty universal: a phallic-shaped shaft with a clitoral attachment that often resembles a cute little animal. More than a hundred rabbit-style vibrators are on the market, available from dozens of different manufacturers, and they all have subtle design differences as well as varied features. The control and battery unit is either at the base of the shaft or in a separate unit attached by a wire. Rabbit-style vibrators can be made of rubber, jelly rubber, PVC, elastomer, TPR, or silicone.

The best rabbit-style vibrators for stimulating the G-spot are those with a curved or bendable shaft. A bendable shaft allows you to control the angle as well as the orbit, because some of these vibes don't just vibrate—they actually circle around inside you. The clitoral attachment also varies from toy to toy. You can choose an animal, which will deliver a light fluttering motion against your clitoris usually with its ears, paws, or antennae. Or if you prefer more pressure against your clit, pick a toy with a more solid attachment—think oval bullet—so you have something firmer to rub against.

CLEANING AND CARING FOR YOUR TOYS

The key to maintaining your toys and having them last a long time is to clean, care for, and store them properly just as you would any other important tools. If you're using rechargeable toys, always follow the charging instructions that come with them. Usually, you must fully charge the toy when you get it home before you use it. Always store your battery-operated toys with the batteries removed, and be sure to change old batteries promptly. There's nothing worse than running out of juice just when you need it most!

In discussing cleaning recommendations, I make an important distinction: You can clean any toy (washing it for hygienic purposes) and you can sterilize some toys depending on what they're made of (so that they may be shared with someone). Educate yourself about what kind of toy you have and what it's made of.

For example, a waterproof toy can be submerged in water, whereas a water-resistant toy won't be damaged if you get some water on it, but it cannot be submerged or soaked. When reading the following, note that no toys with electrical components should be soaked, boiled, or put in the dishwasher. These toys should be wiped down only. After washing, allow toys to air-dry, because drying them with any kind of towel can leave some lint clinging to your toy. When storing your toys, keep them out of direct sunlight, away from heat sources, and in a place with some air circulation but not a lot of moisture. It's best to store them in individual bags: satin or another silky material is ideal for silicone, soft and padded for glass and metal.

Latex, PVC, vinyl, elastomer, TPR, and other soft materials: These can be washed (but not sterilized) with warm water and mild soap or a sex toy cleaner. If you want to share one of these toys, you should cover it with a new condom for each partner.

Silicone: Clean with hot water and antibacterial soap or a sex toy cleaner. Or sanitize them by (1) soaking for a few minutes in a diluted bleach solution of 10 parts water to 1 part bleach (rinse them very well), (2) washing in the top rack of the dishwasher without detergent, or (3) placing in boiling water for about 3 minutes.

Hard plastic: Hard plastics include resin, urethane, PVC (without softeners), and any other solid plastics. Hard plastic toys run the gamut between those that are porous and those that aren't. All of them may be cleaned with warm water and a mild antibacterial soap or a sex toy cleaner. Unless the manufacturer states that the plastic is medical-grade and nonporous, assume that it cannot be sterilized.

Glass: Clean them with warm water and antibacterial soap or a sex toy cleaner. Disinfect them by soaking them in a diluted bleach solution (10:1) or alcohol. If you know the toy is borosilicate glass, you can put it in the top rack of the dishwasher without detergent on a gentle setting to sterilize it.

Aluminum, stainless steel, and other metals: Metal can be cleaned with warm water and antibacterial soap and sterilized with a diluted bleach solution (10:1) or alcohol. Or place it in the top rack of the dishwasher without detergent. Metal toys must be dried completely to prevent rusting and/or corrosion.

A variation of the rabbit style—which I call "phallic with wings"—resembles a traditional phallic vibrator with, well, wings. Imagine a phallic insertable vibe shaped like a hooked finger. About halfway down the shaft it has two small extensions, kind of like wings, which are often textured. When you slide the shaft inside you, the wings rest at your vaginal opening, one stimulating your vulva and clitoris, the other the sensitive perineum.

Curved Double-Action Vibes

You can think of curved double-action vibrators as vibrating wands except they are usually made of silicone. Whereas the rabbit-style vibe is phallic, these tend to more closely resemble wands: They are curvy U, S, and "smile" shapes. Some of them have such a dramatic curve that you can wear them for hands-free fun. If you find that a rabbit-style vibe isn't hitting your G-spot, try one of these. One end goes inside you for targeted G-spot stimulation, and the other end sits externally against your vulva. Compared with a rabbit-style vibrator, the external part of a curved double-action vibe tends to have more surface area and really wraps around the vulva, providing better (and often stronger) vibration for the clitoris. Slide the insertable part in your vagina; once inside, the outer part cups your vulva and clitoris, delivering vibration inside and out.

SAFER SEX

If you're in a monogamous relationship, have tested negative for all sexually transmitted infections—gonorrhea, chlamydia, syphilis, herpes, HPV, hepatitis, and HIV—and regularly have unprotected sex with your partner, you can engage in all the activities in this book with confidence. However, if you aren't monogamous, you and your partner haven't been tested, or you're not sure, then you should practice safer sex. Use barriers to protect yourself and your partner from body fluids, including semen, vaginal fluids, female ejaculate, rectal bacteria, and menstrual blood.

CONDOMS

For vaginal and anal intercourse, use a condom every time. Rather than seeing condoms as inconvenient or disruptive to your lovemaking, make them a positive part of the experience. Take the lead and put the condom on his cock yourself. Or stroke or lick his balls as he slides a condom on. You can also learn to put a condom on with your mouth, which is a sexy way to keep the action going.

Non-lubricated condoms without any bumps, ridges, or other textures on the outside are best for oral sex. You can also try out flavored condoms, which are made for oral sex, to see if there's a flavor you like. If you or your partner is sensitive or allergic to latex, be sure to choose a non-latex condom. If you find that your own saliva dries up or is not enough to lubricate the condom for a smooth and comfortable blow job, apply a little lube to the outside of the condom. Be sure to select a flavored lube or a lube with a taste you don't mind. It's better to use an unlubricated condom because you can control what kind of lube you use and how much.

If your sex toy is made of a porous material—rubber, PVC, vinyl, jelly rubber, or CyberSkin—don't share it with other people unless you put a condom on it first and use a new condom for each new partner. If your sex toy is made of a nonporous material—hard plastic, silicone, acrylic, glass, or metal—you can share it with other people as long as you clean the toy between partners. Follow cleaning guidelines from the toy's manufacturer. You can also cover these toys with a condom and use a new condom for each new partner.

No research has been conducted on female ejaculate and sexually transmitted infections (STIs). From what we know about it, female ejaculatory fluid does not have as high a concentration of sexually transmitted organisms as semen or blood does; however, it is still a body fluid and may contain some amount of organisms. As part of safer sex, you should use condoms, gloves, and barriers if your partner is a female ejaculator.

ORAL DAMS

For safer cunnilingus and analingus, you can purchase a latex dam or dental dam at better sex stores and websites. Dab a little bit of lube on the side that will cover her genitals, then place the square over her entire vulva or anus. Dams are very thin yet durable, so both of you will be able to feel every move and still be protected. A dam is meant for onetime use, so throw it away when you're done.

If you or your partner is sensitive or allergic to latex, or you prefer a different kind of barrier, you can use regular plastic wrap found in any grocery store. Plastic wrap doesn't limit you to a particular size of plastic, like a dam does, but it works the same way a dam does. You can also fit the plastic to her body for hands-free licking.

Another way to create an oral sex barrier is to make one out of a latex or non-latex glove. Take the glove and cut off all the fingers except the thumb. Then cut up the side where the pinky was. Open the glove, slide your tongue in the thumb, and violà—it's like a condom for your tongue! If you are practicing safer sex, you also want to use a latex or non-latex glove for penetration. Be sure to get the proper size glove for your hand, so you have the most sensitivity. Always use a water-based or silicone-based lubricant with a glove to reduce friction and make penetration much more pleasurable.

CHAPTER 5

EROTIC INTERLUDE #1: "THE ABGS"

BY ALISON TYLER

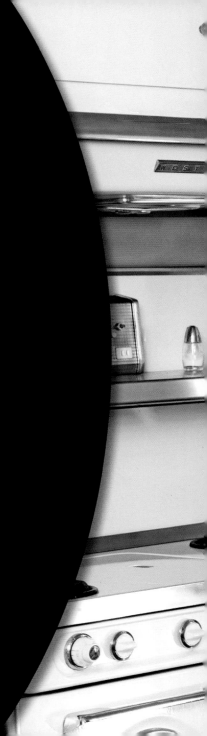

"There's no such thing."

"Come on, baby, you believe in crop circles, don't you?"

"That's different, Dave."

"And I *think* I heard you talk about Area 51 once."

"Stop teasing."

"Max, you put your faith in all sorts of homeopathic mumbo jumbo from tea tree oil to the powers of nux vomica. Why are you so dead set against this?"

"Because you're talking about my body. I know myself inside out. What you're describing doesn't exist. Otherwise, I'd have found it by now."

"I'm not lying to you. I swear."

I looked at him. He had that earnest expression on his face, the one that let me know he wasn't about to stop harassing me unless I allowed him to complete his piece. I sighed, tightened the belt on my silk robe, then settled back against the pillows, waiting for him to continue.

"Look, for a girl who believes in as many whacked-out conspiracy theories as you do . . . "

"Global warming is *not* a conspiracy theory . . . "

"You ought to let me demonstrate my considerable knowledge."

"Oh, that's right. The great Lothario is going to teach me."

"What do you have to lose, Maxine? If I'm wrong, then we've just had sex. And if I'm right, then we've just had fabulous, mind-blowing, call-all-your-girlfriends-and-tell-them-I'm-a-god sex."

He did have a point. Sex with Dave is never a waste of time. He always knows exactly what I need. That didn't mean I had to give in gracefully. I'm stubborn with a capital S.

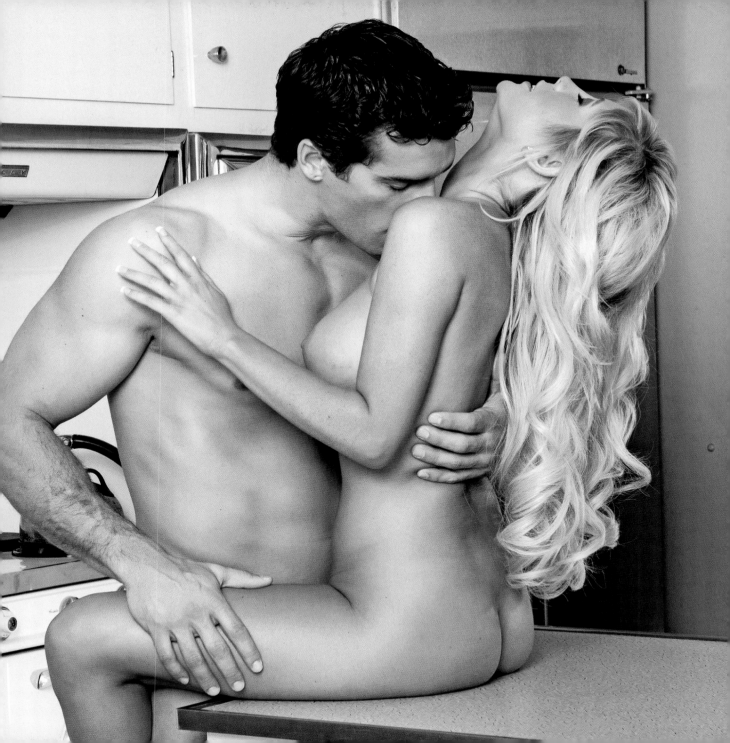

"So what do you want me to do?"

He went into the bathroom and returned with a terry cloth towel.

"I'm not wet, Dave."

"You're going to be."

I watched as he spread the towel out on the bed. Then he said, "Now, lie back, and get comfortable."

I did as he told me. Well, I did the "lie back" part. The "get comfortable" part was more difficult. My nerves jangled, for no real reason at all. "Now what?"

"You don't think the G-spot exists, is that right?"

"Yes, sir."

"So let's start with you're A-spot."

I stared up at the ceiling and frowned. "There's no such thing as an A-spot."

"Says you."

He started undressing. I lifted my head and watched. Dave is built like the rock-climbing, mountain-biking, long-distance-running athlete that he is. The muscles on his arms alone make me happy. Don't get me started on his six-pack . . . He took off his clothes too quickly for my opinion. I enjoy a good striptease every now and again. But Dave was on a mission.

When he was naked, he took off my clothes. That was easy. I was only wearing a robe, after all. Then he started to kiss me until I was breathless. Still, that didn't take my mind off what we were doing. I was so curious to see his plans for the hunt for my G-spot that I was aware of every little nuance, every subtle touch, each tiny sensation. He was doing nothing new, and I started to tell him so.

"Dave—"

"You need a hard O first."

"You're losing me with all this alphabetical bullshit."

"In order to best locate your G-spot, you need one strong climax. Just to get things going."

I opened my mouth to say something flippant, but then shut it again. Who was I to argue with that plan?

"Relax, baby," Dave said, and I closed my eyes and felt him position himself on top of me. "Now, while the G-spot is in the same general location on all women, the rest of the spots are more difficult to pin down. For instance, I'd call this your A-spot," Dave said, tonguing the under curve of my neck.

I have always loved to be touched there, and my man knows that. I tilted my head back, giving him as much access as he could desire. He stroked his fingertips along the hollow of my throat, then kissed me there some more, until I moaned.

"God, that feels good."

As if those words were the cue, he continued down my body, kissing my nipples . . . "Spot B and spot C," he said.

"How can you tell them apart?"

"They're interchangeable."

"That doesn't sound very scientific."

"Shhh."

He licked and sucked on my left nipple while pinching and tweaking my right. I didn't think I was going to make it to spot D if he continued like that. My whole body felt electrified. But Dave's a pro. He seemed to know when my heart started to pound faster, when my pussy started to grow wetter, and he began biting gently along the valley of my stomach until he reached the ring adorning my belly button.

"You're going to say that's my D-spot, aren't you?"

"Bingo."

"Should have been B for Belly Button."

"Semantics," he said, dismissing my critique and licking and tugging gently on the sterling silver ring he'd chosen for me. I thought about the feeling of being pierced under Dave's watch, thought about how he'd fucked me in his truck afterward, and I got wetter still. Dave hadn't told me we were going to a piercing studio that night. He'd driven me to the spot up on Sunset, parked the car, and waited until I realized where we were. He's like that. He plans for occasions, reveals his hand slowly.

With me, things are different. I'm WYSIWYG, as Dave says. What you see is what you fucking get. I'm piss-poor at playing poker. Right now, I couldn't hide the fact that I was growing more aroused by the second.

Thank God we only had to work our way to G—if Grafenberg had been Zafenberg, I'd have passed out from pleasure before we reached a Z-spot.

"E and F are coming up," Dave said, giving me fair warning. My head was spinning. E and F apparently were my nether lips, because Dave pulled them apart, pinching me and making me jump.

"The F-spot better be for Fucking," I hissed.

"What a dirty mouth you have."

"I want your cock in me," I demanded.

"Weren't you a DOS girl before you got a Mac?"

"What the hell does that have to do with sex?"

"You remember how bizarre the commands were, don't you? It was like O for Delete and Y for Save."

"You're about to tell me my F-spot is my clit, isn't it?"

"I'm no doctor," he said with a smile.

Now that he had my lips spread, he could tell exactly how wet I was. I didn't have to look down to tell. I knew my clit was swollen and ready, knew my shaved lips were creamy. I couldn't explain it. But maybe all this talk about what a G-spot orgasm was like had put me in the mood. I felt the callused ball of his thumb roll over my clitoris, and I groaned and started to beat my hips against the towel.

"Calm down, Maxine," Dave whispered. "You don't have to rush."

"I can't calm down," I told him honestly. "Not when you touch me like that."

"Like this?"

His thumb ran over my clit again, and then he pressed hard against me. Dave touches me exactly the way I touch myself when I'm alone. I've never been with a lover like him before. He seems to read my body as if he's working his own. The way he stroked me now took me to the very edge. He tricked his fingertips around my clit, then ran his thumb over and over that hot spot, alternating pressure until I shuddered and came.

A hard O. That's exactly what I had.

"Good girl," he said, bending down to lick me. I couldn't take the pressure so soon, and I pushed him away from my pussy. Dave positioned himself down on the mattress. When he gazed up my body, I saw the gloss of my pleasure on his lips, and a shiver flickered through me. He looked so handsome like that, in between my thighs. He looked even sexier when he said, "I'm going to show you your G-spot now."

"Fine." As I said the word, I wished I could take it back. I didn't sound grateful or pleased at all. My tone was skeptical.

"You still don't believe me, do you?"

"I believe you believe it," I said, knowing I sounded exactly the way people talk to folks who claim to have been taken off by aliens.

"I'm not stopping until you do."

"Stopping what?"

"This."

And then he was in me—not with his cock, but with his hand. I was surprised at the way he seemed to zone exactly in on one particular region, completely forgoing my clit. He slid in his fingers and began to curl them against the inner wall of my body, as if he were beckoning someone closer. The sensation crept up on me slowly, stealthily, and then suddenly I said, "I think I have to pee."

"It'll pass."

"If you don't want this to be the Wet Spot for real, you should stop."

"Trust me."

I glared at him. But he was right. In seconds that sensation passed, replaced instead by something better, something bigger . . .

"Jesus."

"Ah hah. I hit it didn't I? On the first try, too." He was smug.

"I—I . . . "

"Don't tell me you still don't believe."

"I mean, I . . . "

"I'll stop if you don't admit it." The opposite of the threat he'd issued only moments before. But this was a threat I took seriously. I would have told him I believed in fairies, Santa Claus, the Easter Bunny, if he promised to continue.

"Don't stop."

"So . . . "

"Oh, God, don't stop."

He kept stroking, or beckoning. He kept *come-hithering* until I knew I was going to be coming, too. I couldn't believe it. I never come a second time so quickly after a first. But I could tell from the way my body was reacting that I was right on the brink once more.

"How did you know? How are you doing that?" I was stammering, stuttering, hardly able to speak.

Dave pulled out his hand.

"Nooooo!"

"Wait . . . "

And then he was poised on his gorgeous arms over my body, and his cock, his lovely cock that has the slightest of upward curves, was in me, deep in me, pressing against that same dreamy spot.

"Jesus."

"You already said that."

"Oh, Dave."

The smile was in his eyes now. He loves when I call his name out during sex.

"You like that, Max?"

I couldn't respond. The way his cock kept touching that spot inside of me was something I'd never felt before.

Like wasn't the right word. But I couldn't spend any time thinking of the right word. All I could manage was, "Yeah."

"I do, too." He was fucking me harder now, but focused, with each stroke landing exactly on that spot. I couldn't speak anymore, couldn't think anymore. All I could do was wrap my thighs around my man and hold on for the ride.

He'd been teasing me with the A-F spots. I knew that. I understood. But the G-spot was real. The G-spot was my new best friend. The G-spot was the only thing that mattered.

Dave got that look in his eyes that lets me know he is close. I sucked in my breath, and he pounded into me, hitting harder and faster against that same spot until I moaned, "I'm coming. Baby, I'm coming."

My man lowered his head and came with me. A hard O doesn't even begin to describe what we shared. They'd have to make up a new word for it.

"Oh, wow," I sighed after. "Oh, man. Oh, Dave."

"Did I make a believer out of you?"

I nodded.

"Wait 'til I show you your Q-spot."

I started to open my mouth, to tell him there was no such thing, and then I thought of the orgasm I'd just had. Who was I to argue?

ALISON TYLER is the author of twenty-five naughty novels and the editor of more than fifty erotic anthologies, most recently *Alison's Wonderland* and *With This Ring I Thee Bed* (both published by Harlequin Spice). Visit her at www.alisontyler.com.

CHAPTER 6

FROM DIGITS TO DILDOS: PARTNERED G-SPOT STIMULATION WITH FINGERS AND TOYS

Orgasms with clitoral stimulation are delightfully sharp, intense, and usually prompt. When my clit is stimulated but the G-spot is the focus, I know it will take longer and require much more energy from both my partner and me. Clitoral stimulation is like a gasp or breathy moan, while adding lots of G-spot stimulation is a gritty, animalistic, hungry, growling roar. I know my orgasm will be a significantly larger release, and that post-orgasmic glow will be that much more intimate—whether I'm solo or with a partner.

—Regina

If you want to find and stimulate your partner's G-spot, your fingers really are the best tools for the job. They're sensitive, flexible, and versatile. Make sure you have clean, short, well-filed nails before you start your exploration; if you're concerned about your nails being less than perfect, slip on a latex or nitrile glove.

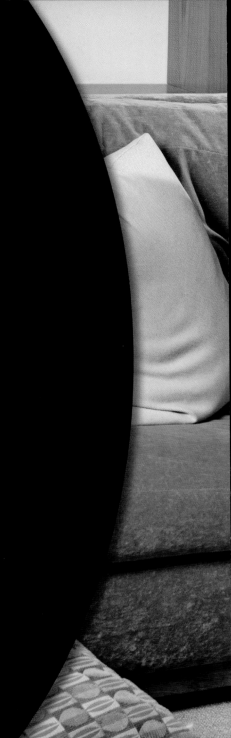

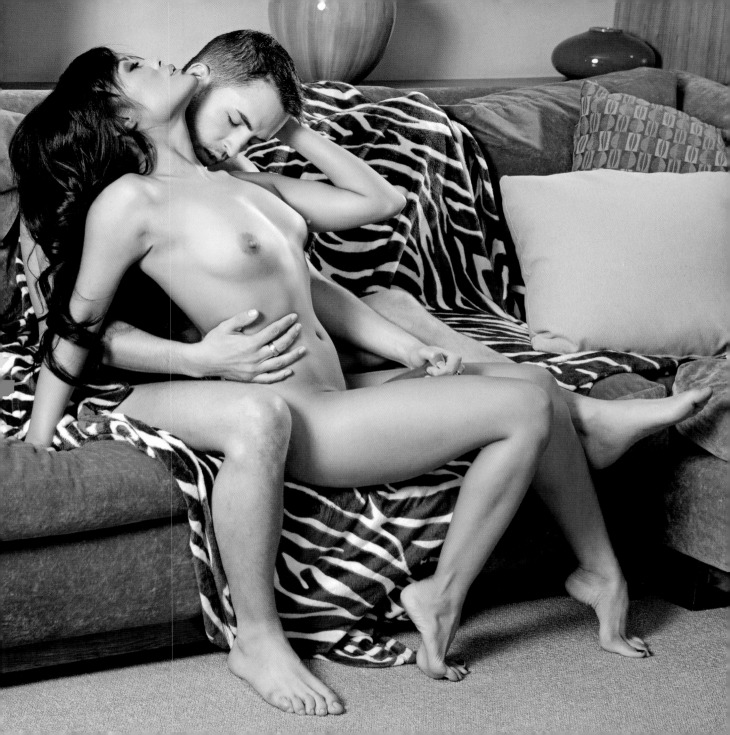

LET YOUR FINGERS DO THE FINDING

1. Ask your partner to lie on her back with her legs spread. You may want to put a pillow under her butt. Being face to face in the beginning is best for kissing, communication, and easy access to lots of hot spots.

2. Start with a nice round of oral sex, manual stimulation, or whatever gets her in the mood.

3. Once she feels warmed up, slide your well-lubed forefinger inside her vagina. Remember to continue to stimulate her clit with your other hand, or she can do it with her own hand or a vibrator.

4. Run your finger along the front wall of her vagina as you slide it slowly in and out. You're not going to try anything fancy at first, just get used to how she feels, get the juices flowing, and build her arousal.

5. When she's ready, add some lube and your middle finger.

6. Feel on the front wall for a wrinkly, ridged area with your fingers. Press on it gently and ask her how it feels; continue to press in different places and let her guide you while you're inside her.

7. Begin some long strokes with your fingers in and out while pressing upward. Longer strokes will let you cover as much surface area as you can, which is helpful in the beginning to let you both pinpoint that sensitive area on the front wall: the G-spot. These strokes will also fuel her arousal.

8. Apply more pressure on the front wall as you move your fingers in and out.

9. When you're confident you've located her G-spot and you're both ready, remember that a light touch won't do much for the G-spot. You want to strive for deliberate, direct, firm pressure. You're stimulating the sponge on the other side of the vaginal wall, which is why pressure, rather than gentle strokes, works best.

10. As with other kinds of stimulation, the key is to build the intensity—don't go too hard too quickly. Communicate with your partner and see what feels best for her.

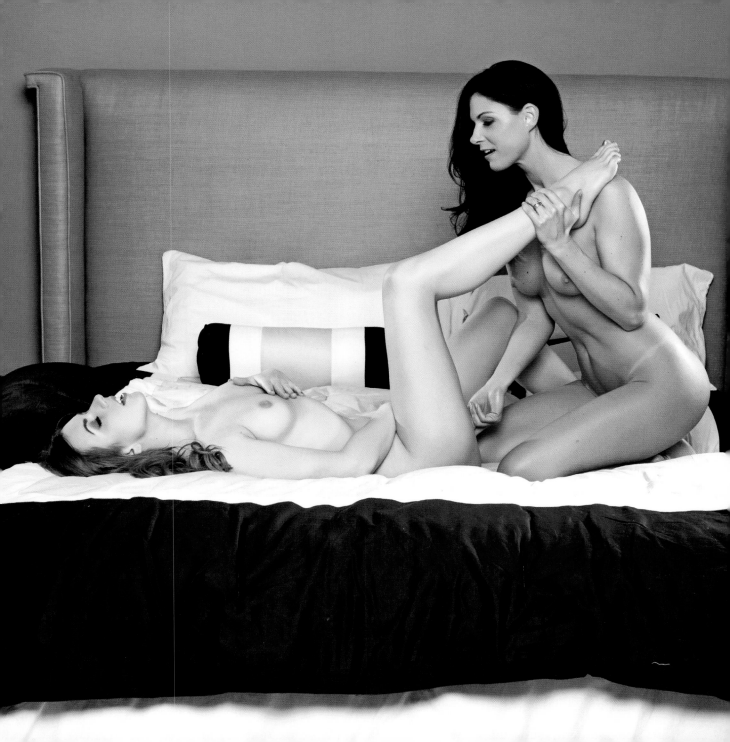

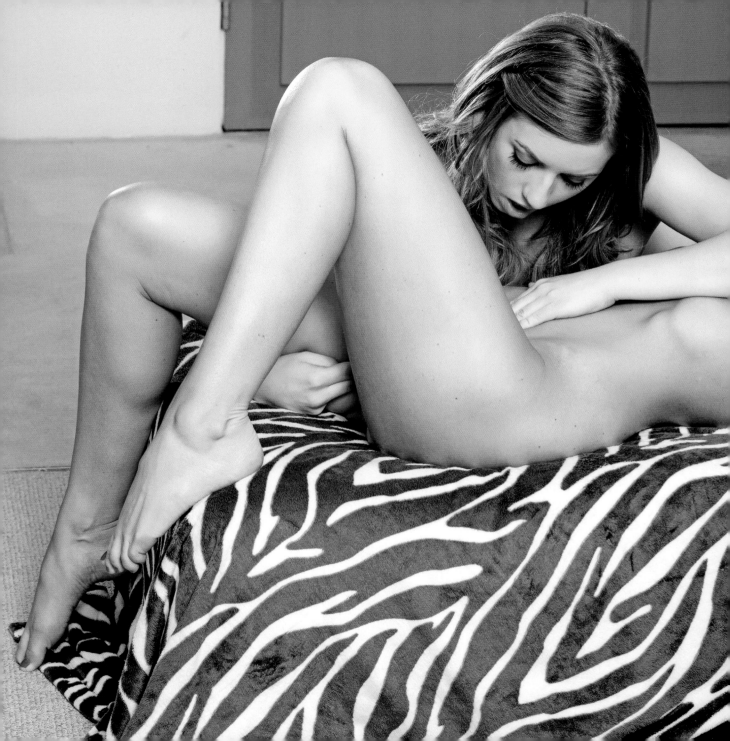

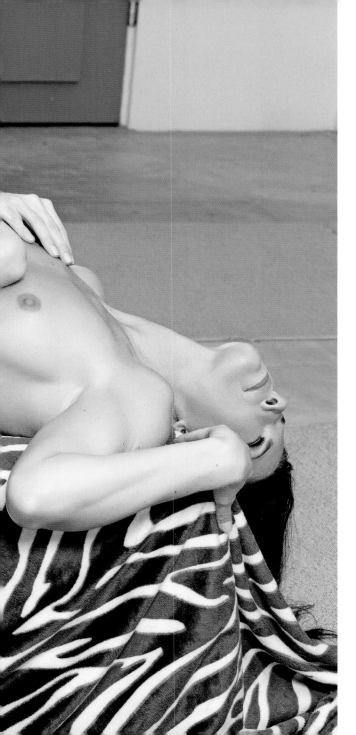

DIFFERENT STROKES FOR DIFFERENT FOLKS

Experiment with different finger techniques, varying the amount of movement, pressure, or both on the G-spot.

Use long strokes, applying an equal amount of pressure and movement, and see how she responds. Some women want you to go all the way in and come nearly all the way out, especially if the entire front wall of the vagina is sensitive and it's not limited to just one spot.

If you can reach her clitoral hood with your thumb while your fingers are inside her vagina, experiment with this trick. Place your thumb on her clitoral hood and stroke downward over the hood with the pad of your thumb as you press and pull inside with your two fingers.

Try this classic G-spot technique: Bend your fingers slightly, like you're trying to hook something with them. Keep applying pressure but decrease the amount of movement. Imagine you're making a "come here" motion with your fingers, aiming toward the front of her body.

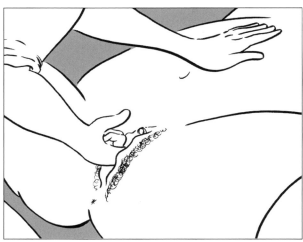

Shorten your strokes, and bring the curve of your fingers toward yourself as if you're trying to pull something out of her; some people also describe this as a kind of digging motion. As you do this, put your other hand at the pubic hairline above the pubic mound and press downward; some people say this feels like you're hitting the spot from both sides.

Another option is to focus almost entirely on the pressure, decreasing the amount of movement. Continue the come here technique with your fingers, but make the pulling motion much more subtle (with very little in-and-out motion), and apply more pressure upward. Or you can alternate pressure with each finger; imagine your fingers are "walking" inside her.

While you're so diligently focused on the G-spot, don't forget about the clitoris. Some women prefer G-spot stimulation by itself, whereas others appreciate both at once. Because all the nerves and tissues are connected, they play off one another, helping stimulate the entire area.

ANGLING FOR POSITION

At some stage in your finger play, your partner may want to change positions. On her hands and knees, with her head and shoulders up or down, and with you behind her in Doggie-Style position, her body is angled perfectly for your fingers to easily hit the front wall of her vagina and her G-spot. This change of angle may also help increase the amount of pressure you can apply, which for some women makes all the difference.

Or you can lie on your back and have your partner straddle you and ride your fingers from above. She can shift her hips to change the angle of penetration, plus you'll be face to face for easy communication.

With your partner in these new positions, experiment again with how much pressure, penetration, and movement she likes—ask her which techniques feel the best to her. If she wants to feel fuller, you can insert more fingers.

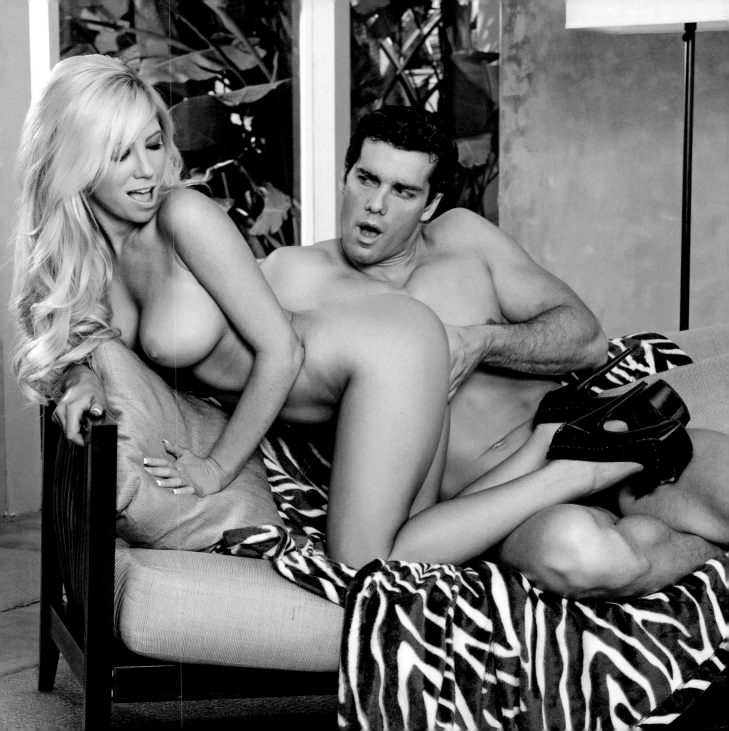

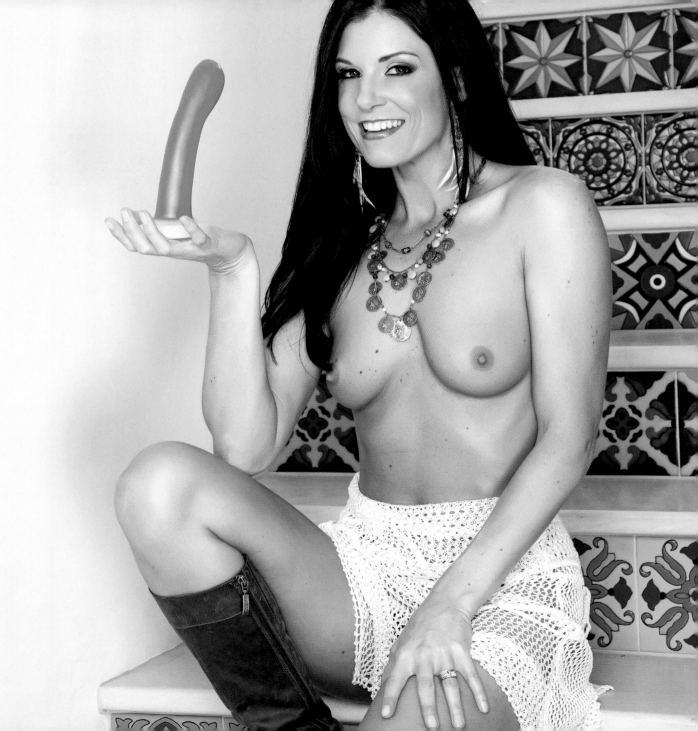

PLAYING WITH TOYS: MY PICKS FOR PARTNERED PLAY

As we've already discussed, sex toys—vibrators, dildos, and wands—are great tools for G-spot exploration, and they are definitely not just for solo play. Toys make a fabulous addition to your partnered sex life. It's a good idea to warm up with cunnilingus, manual stimulation, or penetration with fingers before introducing a toy to the mix. As you read in chapter 4, you can find a wide variety of sex toys on the market, many of them designed specifically for the G-spot. Here are some of my top picks and some advice about how to use them for maximum G-spot fireworks.

DELICIOUS DILDO: RAQUEL BY VIXEN CREATIONS

If you're looking for a toy made of a softer material, then my choice is Raquel, which has a slightly bulbous head that makes it perfect for G-spot stimulation. This 7-inch (17.5 cm) dildo is made of VixSkin, a unique blend of top-quality silicone that combines a firm inner core with a softer outer layer to give it an unbeatable fleshlike feeling. Because it's silicone, it warms to body temperature, plus it's flexible enough to bend a little bit inside you to get just the right angle.

Coat the dildo with your favorite water-based lube (or cover the dildo with a condom to use a silicone lube), then grab hold of it at the base and slide it inside your partner. Press it up toward her G-spot and use that same kind of pulling motion you did with your fingers.

WONDEROUS WAND: NJOY PURE WAND

The Pure Wand by Njoy has quite a fan club—women rave about this stainless steel smile-shaped wand, and some think it is *the* best G-spot toy on the market. Because it's made of metal, it is rock hard and feels weighty when you hold it in your hands, both qualities that work really well for G-spot stimulation. The design is not only aesthetically pleasing but also very functional: The curved bulbous ends stimulate the G-spot well, and they make great handles to hold on to for either solo or partnered play. For women who want something more generous, try Pure Wand's less curved, larger cousin, the Eleven.

1. Ask your partner to lie on her back with her butt scooted down to the edge of the bed.

2. Stand in front of her at the edge of the bed as she bends her knees and rests her feet on your abdomen. I call this the Flying Missionary position. This position has many of the pluses of the standard Missionary position—it's good for eye contact, communication, and kissing. A woman can take a more active role in the penetration, using her feet for leverage to push off your body, and both partners have a great view of each other's bodies.

3. Warm her up with some oral sex or manual stimulation.

4. When she's ready, slide the well-lubed Pure Wand inside her.

5. Start with the smaller end and aim the curve upward, toward the front of her body to stimulate her G-spot. She should feel the ball on the end of the toy press against her G-spot as the toy moves in and out of her.

6. Make sure the curve and ball are rubbing against her front wall. Remember, this toy has zero flexibility, so it really has to line up in just the right way inside her. If she wants, you can move up to the larger end.

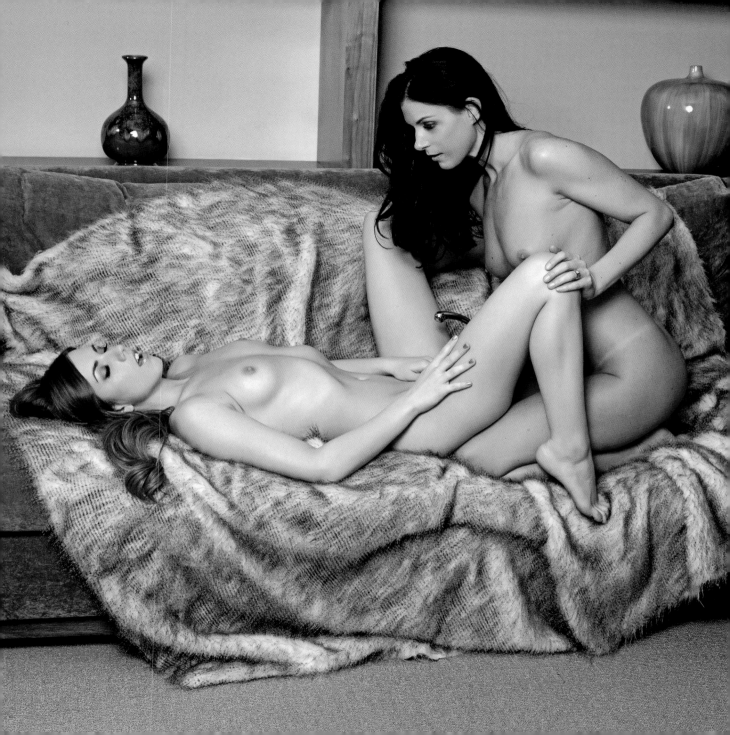

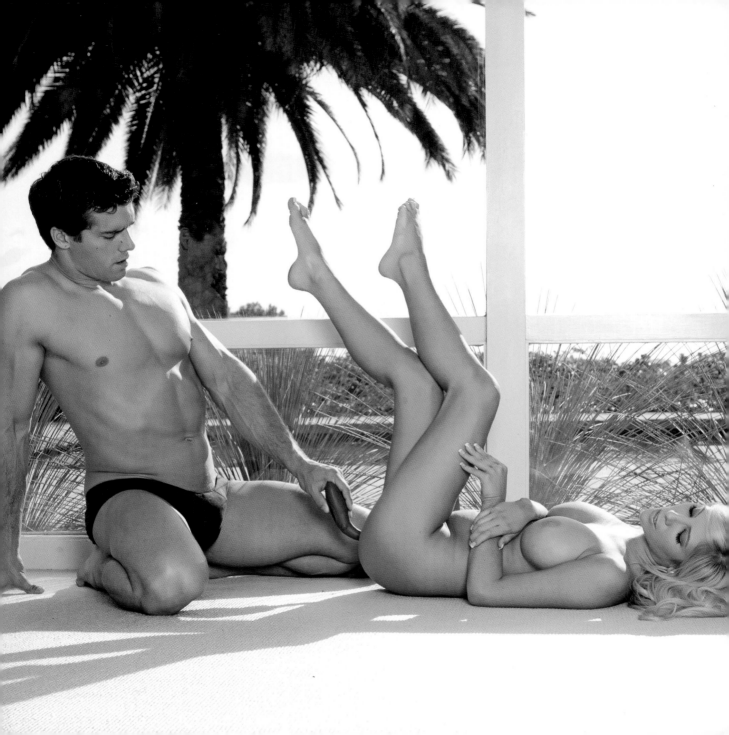

DELIGHTFUL DUAL-ACTION: JE JOUE G-KI

Made of silicone-covered hard plastic, the G-Ki by Je Joue is part of the newest wave in sex toys with smart design and technology. The G-Ki, a curved insertable vibrator, boasts top-notch design and construction, along with five different speeds and five different vibration patterns. In addition, the curve of the toy is adjustable at two different points so you can change it to get the perfect angle or even transform it into a dual-action vibrator.

1. I recommend that you begin with the G-Ki in its original position (in other words, don't adjust the curve at either point yet).

2. Lube the end that is opposite the control panel and slide it inside her.

3. Ask if she wants to feel more vibration or a different pattern, and experiment with those options.

4. As you use the familiar pulling motion to move the toy in and out of her, ask her if she wants to try a more dramatic curve. If she does, take the toy out of her, press and hold the button with three raised dots (the button near the head or insertable part of the toy), bend the toy, then take your finger off the button. This will increase the angle of the curve.

5. Re-lube it, slide it back in her, and ask how that feels. Because G-Ki is a vibrating toy, you may need less in-and-out motion; opt for pressure and a more subtle motion, letting the toy stay in contact with the G-spot.

6. If you'd like to adjust the other section of the toy, press and hold the button with five raised dots (the button closer to the on/off buttons), adjust the toy, then release the button. This will turn it from a smile shape to a J shape, so that the external part vibrates against her clitoris when the other end is inside.

VIRTUOUS VIBRATOR: FUN FACTORY'S DELIGHT

The Delight made by Fun Factory is an S-shaped vibrating toy. One end of the S is for insertion and the other end makes a convenient handle. Just as you did with your fingers, you want to experiment with different levels of pressure and motion when using this toy. Your partner may like long strokes that let the toy's bulbous head stimulate her G-spot on the way in and out. She may prefer shorter strokes that provide a fairly constant pressure on her G-spot with less movement. As you slide the toy inside your partner, the exterior part of it (the middle of the S shape) rubs and vibrates against her vulva and clitoris, creating simultaneous external clitoral stimulation and internal G-spot stimulation.

⟲TRISTAN'S TIPS

This toy comes in one size, and it's not flexible (or adjustable like the G-Ki). It fits each woman differently, and the Delight may not line up in just the right way for your partner to achieve both kinds of stimulation at once. If that's the case, treat it as a vibrating G-spot dildo, and stimulate her clitoris with your hand, her hand, or another vibrator.

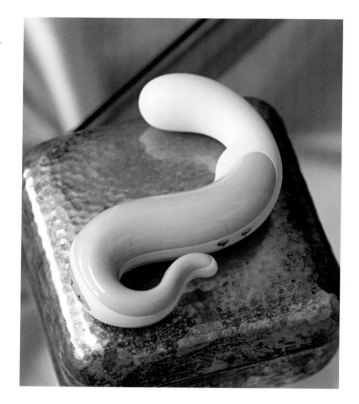

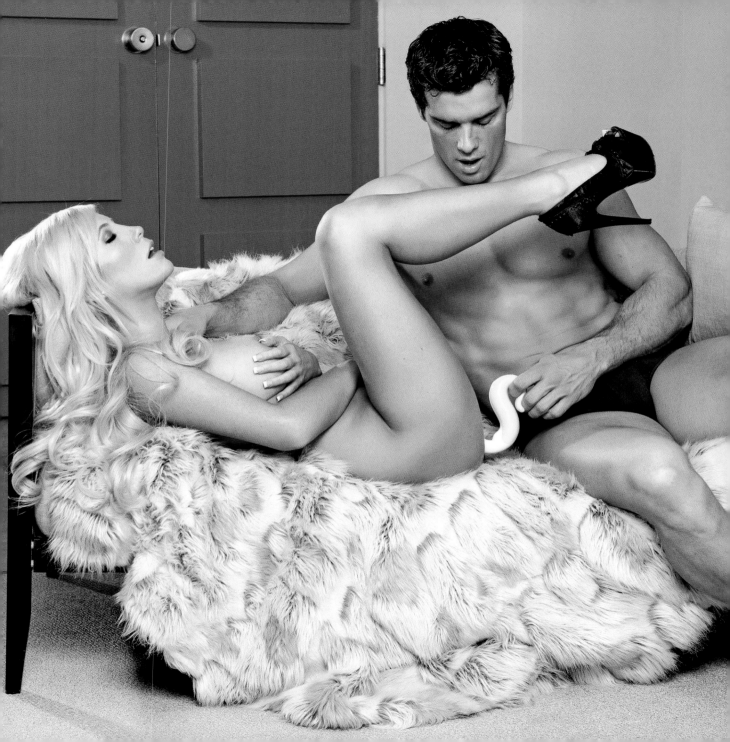

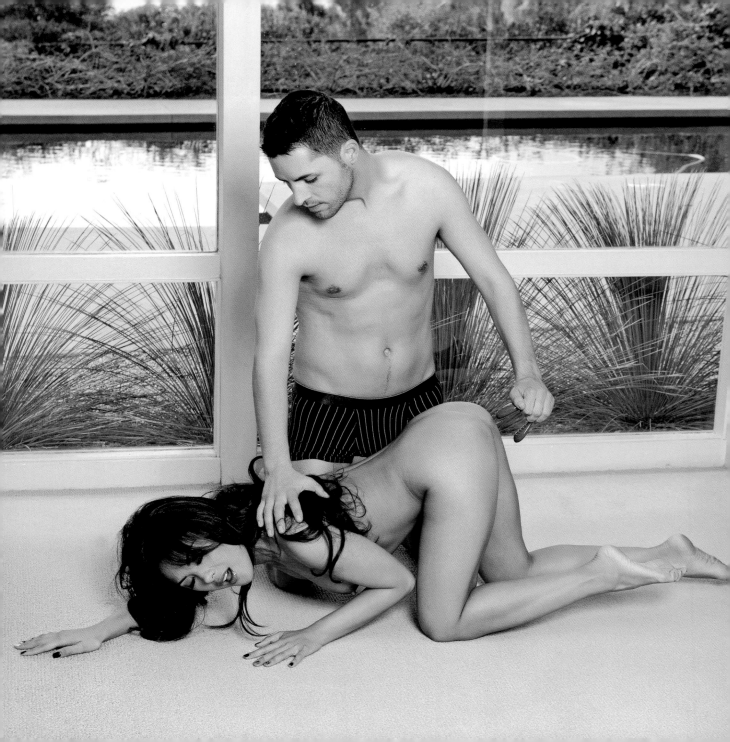

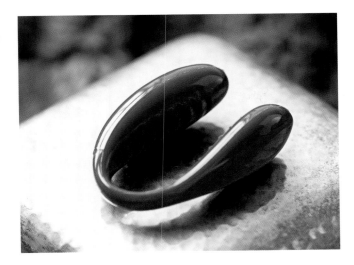

WICKEDLY WEARABLE: THE WE-VIBE II

The We-Vibe II is a unique dual-action vibrator. Made of silicone, rechargeable, and waterproof, it delivers simultaneous clitoral and G-spot stimulation. The U-shaped We-Vibe II resembles a soft pair of tongs with one slimmer end and one slightly wider end. One of the great things about the We-Vibe II is that it's so slim you can wear it during intercourse, and it doesn't get in the way of penetration—in fact, it was designed to be used during penetration.

1. Slide the slimmer end inside her vagina, and as you do so, the wider end hugs the entire vulva.

2. With every thrust of your fingers, dildo, or penis, the internal portion rubs and vibrates right against the G-spot, while the wider, external end vibrates against the clitoris.

3. Give yourself and your partner time to get used to the feeling—it will be a new sensation to have something vibrating inside during intercourse. Because it's quite slim, most men don't feel that it's in the way during intercourse, although they do feel the vibration—which is a good thing!

4. Try the We-Vibe II during Doggie Style or standing position. The force of your thrusting should press the internal part of the toy right against her G-spot.

GETTING IT GOOD: RECEIVING G-SPOT STIMULATION

As noted previously, when your G-spot is stimulated, you may feel like you have to pee. For some women, the urge to pee may be uncomfortable or irritating, or it may make them anxious. For others, when they're aroused and the entire genital region is stimulated and sensitive, the feeling registers as pleasure. It's a common feeling, but you've got to let go of the fear that you're going to pee. Tensing your PC muscles—the muscles that stop the flow of urine—is a common and sometimes automatic response, but it's the opposite of what you want to be doing.

Take some deep breaths and try to relax into the feeling. Try to focus on all the stimulation, rather than your anxiety, and see if that helps transform the sensations you're feeling. Your response to G-spot stimulation can also change. Sometimes G-spot pressure feels great, orgasmic, out of this world; other times, the G-spot feels overly sensitive or too delicate for pressure, or stimulating it just doesn't feel good.

Communicating with your partner during sex is important, especially when trying out a new technique, toy, or position. I know it can feel intimidating, but muster the courage to open your mouth. This is the time to be specific—a little to the left, harder, not so fast. Whatever it is you want to say, be ready to give your partner details and directions. If you feel comfortable doing so, show your partner how you like to use a toy. Demonstrate the angle that works, or how far inside you like it. The more information and feedback you give your partner, the more enjoyable the experience will be for both of you.

CHAPTER 7

POSITIONS TO HIT THE SPOT: INTERCOURSE AND G-SPOT STIMULATION

I don't have G-spot orgasms very often, but when I do it's just as exciting for me as it is for my partner. As with any orgasm, I can feel it coming from afar, like a train coming down the tracks. Then it builds and builds, getting closer . . . closer . . . closer until my whole body is washed over with complete and absolute joy and ecstasy. I point my toes, grab on to whatever is closest with my hands, and scream loudly until it is one long, steady note like an opera singer. Unfortunately for me, I clinch my pelvic muscles so tight when I'm coming that I squeeze out whoever is inside of me!

—Angela

As I've said previously, vaginal intercourse is not necessarily the best way to stimulate your G-spot. In fact, women who primarily have only intercourse often say they can't find their G-spots—and that's because they haven't tried other kinds of stimulation, such as using fingers and toys. When a man with an average-size penis penetrates your vagina, he can slide right past your G-spot, because it's just 1 inch (2.5 cm) or so inside. Because the G-spot is located behind the front wall of the vagina, body position and the angle of penetration matter a great deal.

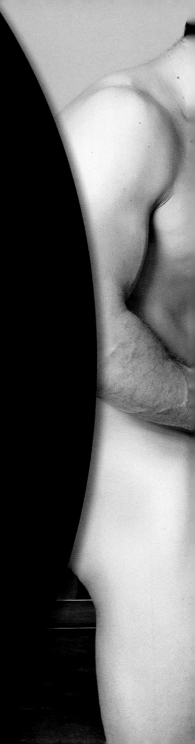

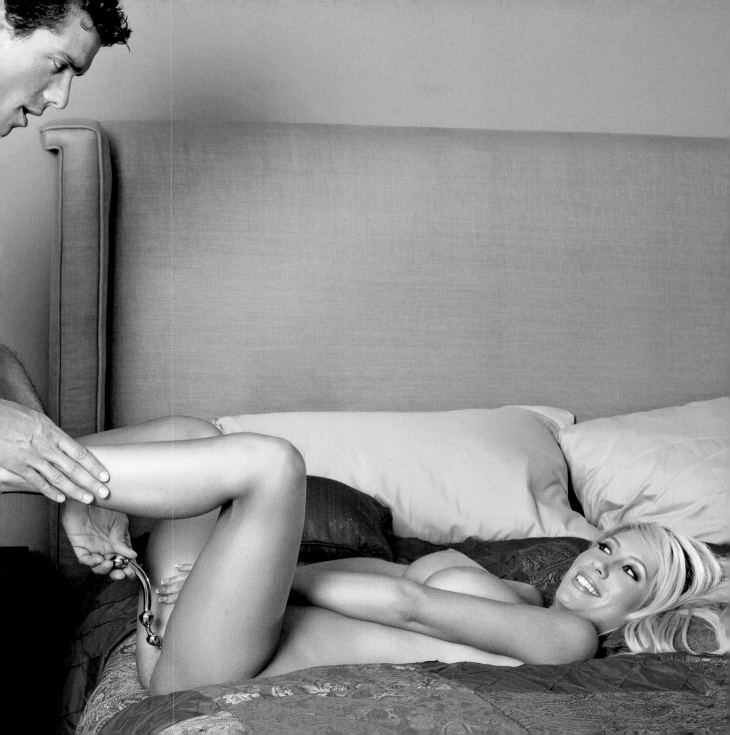

To maximize your chances for targeted G-spot stimulation, explore different positions that accomplish one or more of the following:

- Angle your bodies so his penis (or her dildo) is hitting the front wall of your vagina.

- Allow good leverage and thrusting power, so your partner can put strong pressure on the G-spot.

- Facilitate shallower, shorter strokes and more frequent contact of the head of the penis or dildo with the G-spot.

Throughout this chapter, I discuss positions for vaginal intercourse with a penis, but all of them work just as well during strap-on sex. Feel free to substitute "dildo" for "penis" (and "she" for "he," if you like)—the instructions and benefits are essentially the same. When it's helpful, I also give specific tips about certain positions for strap-on users.

DOGGIE STYLE

In Doggie-Style position, you get on your hands and knees and your partner enters you from behind.

1. If you put your head and shoulders down, with your butt up, your body is at an ideal angle for easy access to your G-spot.

2. As he enters you from behind, his penis will naturally aim downward slightly, hitting the front wall of your vagina.

3. As he moves in and out, the head of his penis can push into the G-spot.

4. If your partner wears a strap-on, make sure the curve of the dildo is aimed toward the front of your body.

5. For added stimulation in Doggie-Style position, your partner can slip a well-lubed finger inside your ass.

FLYING DOGGIE

This position gives your partner more thrusting power, which can mean more intense stimulation for the G-spot. Flying Doggie depends a lot on the height of your bed and your partner, so it definitely won't work for everyone. It's good for partners with knee problems or those who feel they sink into the bed too much and can't get enough leverage for proper thrusting.

1. Begin in Doggie-Style position, but move so your feet are at the edge of the bed. Your partner stands behind you, and now you're in Flying Doggie position.

2. It's ideal if he enters you from slightly above, so his penis can make good contact with your G-spot.

3. For strap-on sex, the person wearing the strap-on can develop good control and rhythm in Flying Doggie position.

4. To kick this position up a notch, wear the We-Vibe II vibrator mentioned earlier.

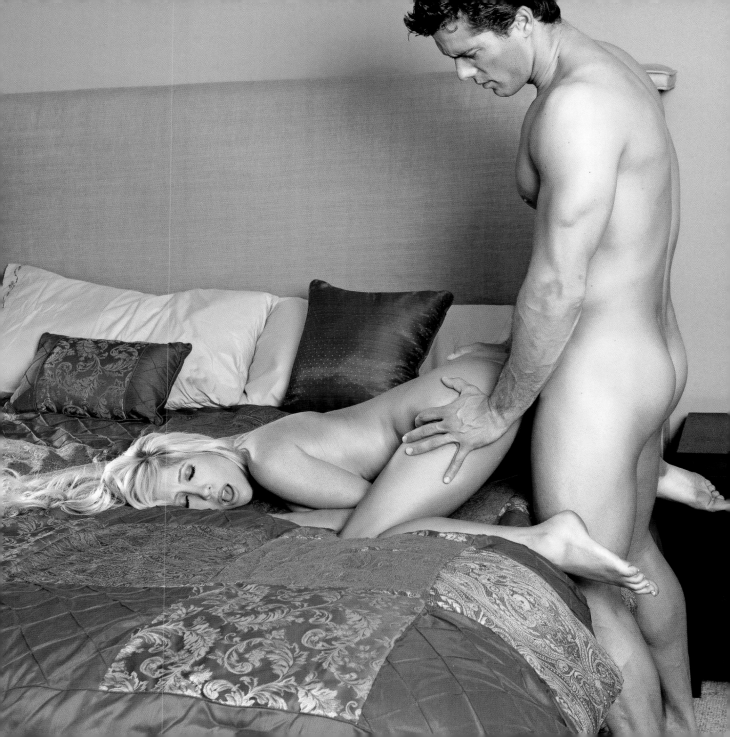

STALLION

In Stallion (which can also be called Standing Doggie), you're off the bed. Stallion has all the benefits of Doggie Style with more power, because he has full leverage to thrust with his hips and legs. His pelvic movements push his penis into your G-spot, creating more vigorous movement and pressure on it than occurs in other positions. If you feel too much strain on your knees in Doggie positions, this is a better option for you. For some couples, this may simply work better than Doggie Style or Flying Doggie because of their sizes and heights.

1. Stand with your legs apart, then bend forward at the waist and lean on the bed (or another piece of furniture) as your partner stands behind you.

2. If he can position his hips slightly higher than yours, he can better stimulate your G-spot.

3. Take Stallion to the next level by placing a mirror in front of you so you can both watch the action.

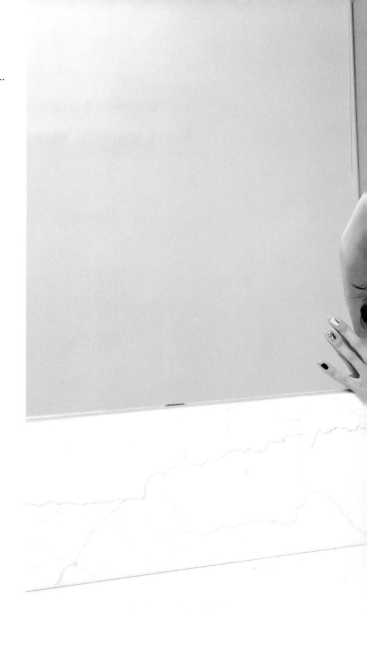

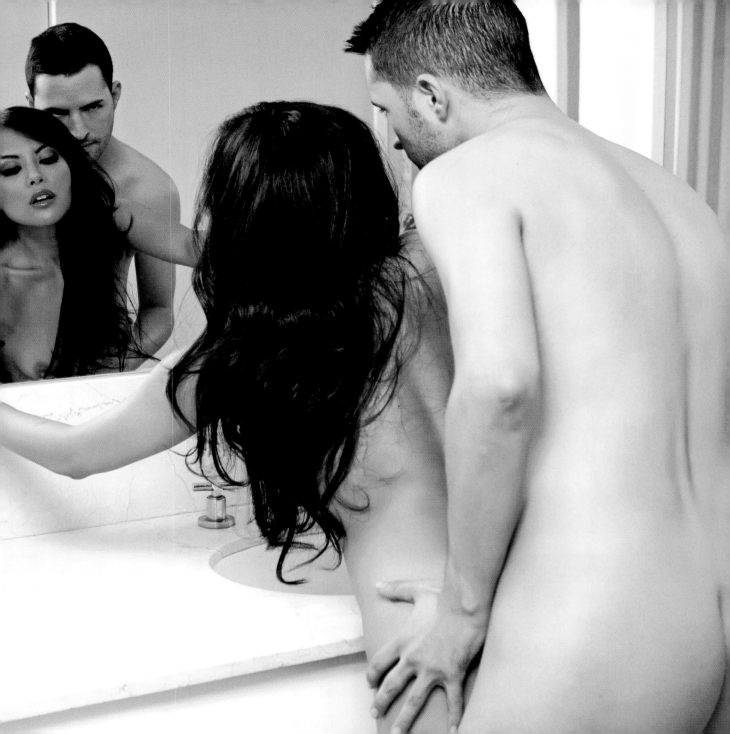

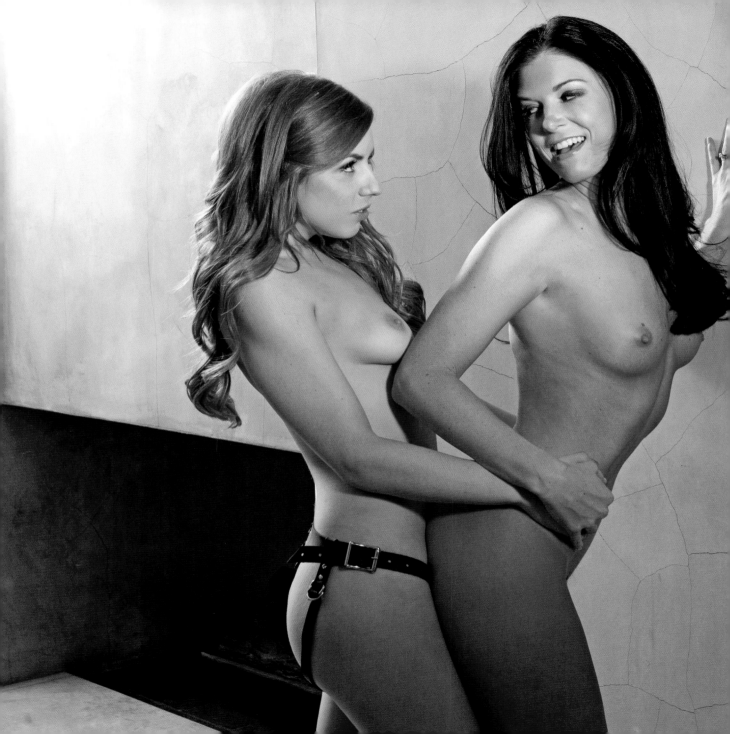

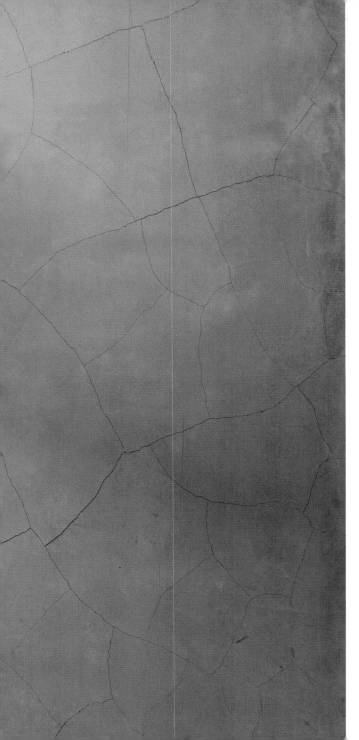

STANDING

If you like Doggie-Style position, but don't like to be bent over or you want your bodies to be closer, I recommend Standing position. He can put his weight behind his thrusting, creating lots of pressure against the front wall of your vagina and G-spot. I don't need to do a lot of explaining for this one: You stand, he stands behind you, and you adjust so you're both comfortable and he has some thrusting power. Obviously, the success of this position depends on your heights and how your bodies line up. But it can give you more skin-to-skin contact, and if the stars (and the two of you) align correctly, some solid G-spot stimulation.

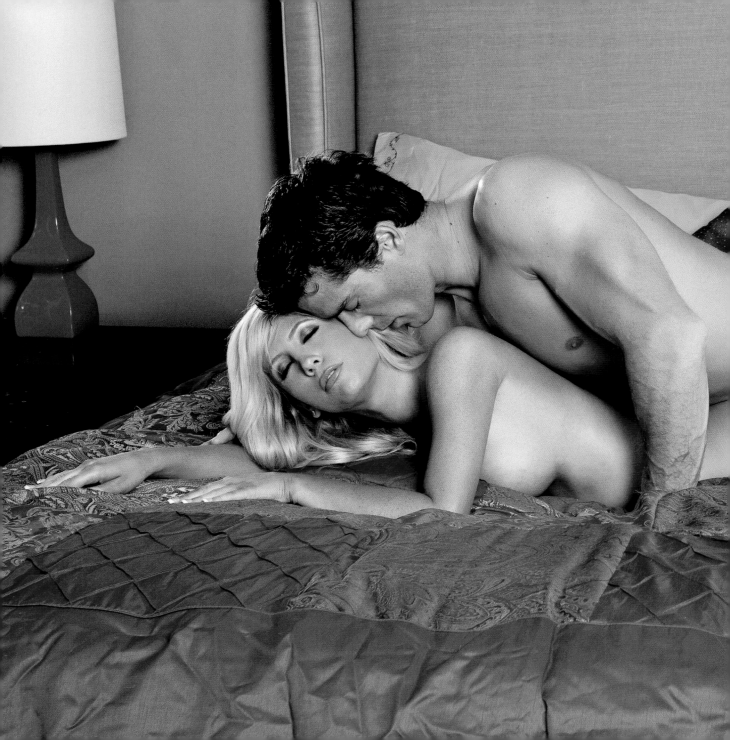

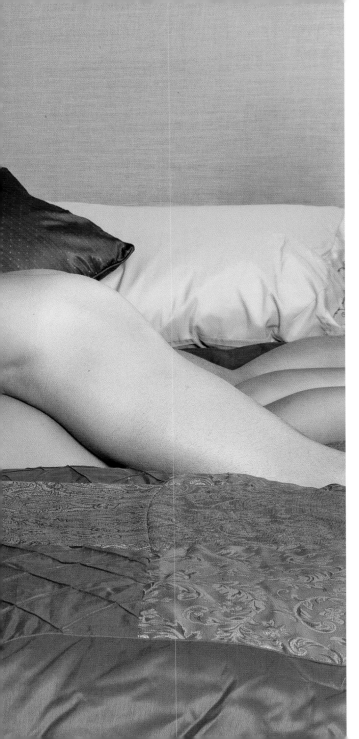

HORIZONTAL TAILGATE

In Horizontal Tailgate position, you lie on your stomach and your partner lies almost completely on top of you. His weight on top of you will add to the deep pressure on your G-spot. I coined the name for this position based on a surfing term: *Tailgating* means to paddle out into the ocean on your surfboard to catch a wave or follow someone else. This is a very intimate position that offers many of the pros of Doggie-Style positions with more skin-to-skin contact and closeness.

1. As he enters you from behind, you can part your legs or tip your hips slightly up toward your partner to make the initial insertion easier.

2. Once he's inside you, he leans all the way forward so that he's lying on top of you.

3. Unlike in Doggie Style, he can't do a lot of deep or powerful thrusting in Horizontal Tailgate, but the angle this position creates can be just as good if not better.

4. He should aim to make small rocking movements.

5. Have more fun in Horizontal Tailgate: He can whisper dirty things in your ear.

YAB-YUM

Yab-Yum is a classic Tantric sex position in which one partner sits in the other partner's lap and they face each other. The man sits with his legs loosely crossed and the woman sits in his lap with her legs wrapped around his waist and torso. The angle of your bodies affords good G-spot contact. He can use firm pillows under his thighs if he needs more support for his legs. If it's not comfortable for him to keep his legs crossed, he can stretch them out in front of him. If he needs back support, he can lean against the wall or the headboard of the bed.

1. As you get into his lap, you can rise up slightly on your knees, he can hold the base of his penis to assist you, and you can slowly ease down onto it. You shouldn't feel any tension or strain; if you do, adjust yourselves so that you can comfortably sink into the position.

2. Look into each other's eyes, and take advantage of the closeness this position affords you.

3. Yab-Yum uses a rocking motion rather than vigorous thrusting. However, because of the angle of your bodies, you can achieve firm pressure on the G-spot.

4. A sitting position such as this one can be trickier for strap-on sex; you may need to adjust where the harness and dildo sit on your body to make this one work for you.

5. Add a twist to this position by synchronizing your breathing with that of your partner. Begin by inhaling and exhaling at the same time. This will bring your awareness to your breath and the connection between you. Focus on the breath and the movement of your bodies; see how your rhythm changes together.

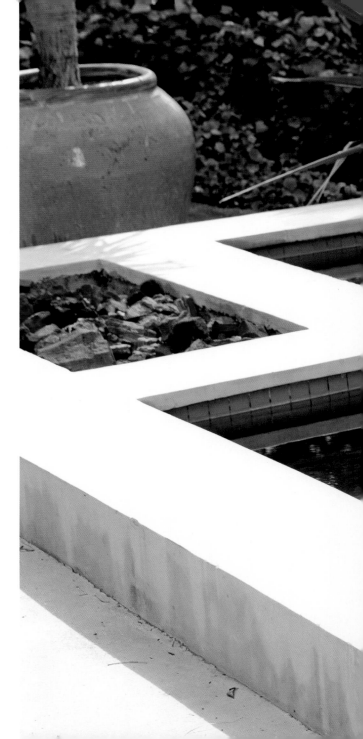

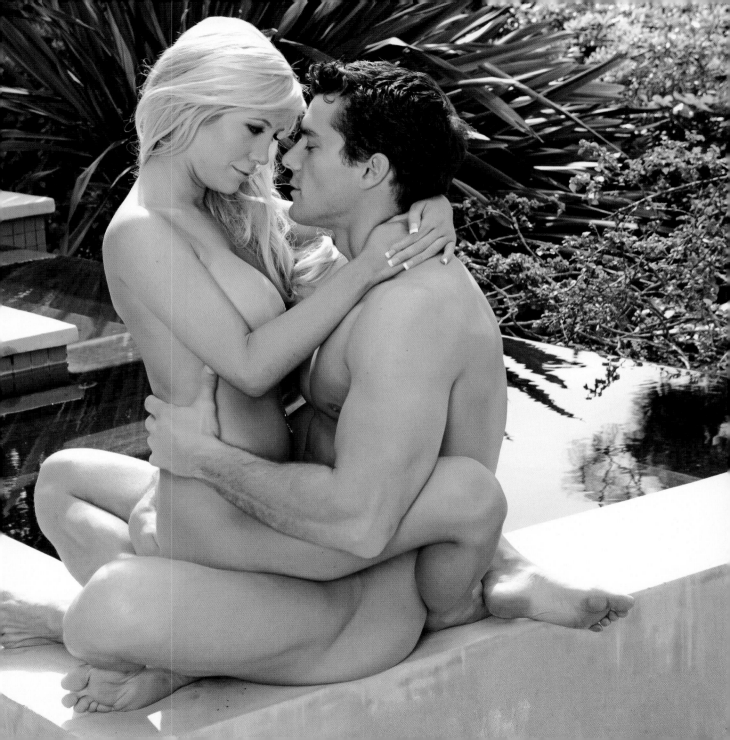

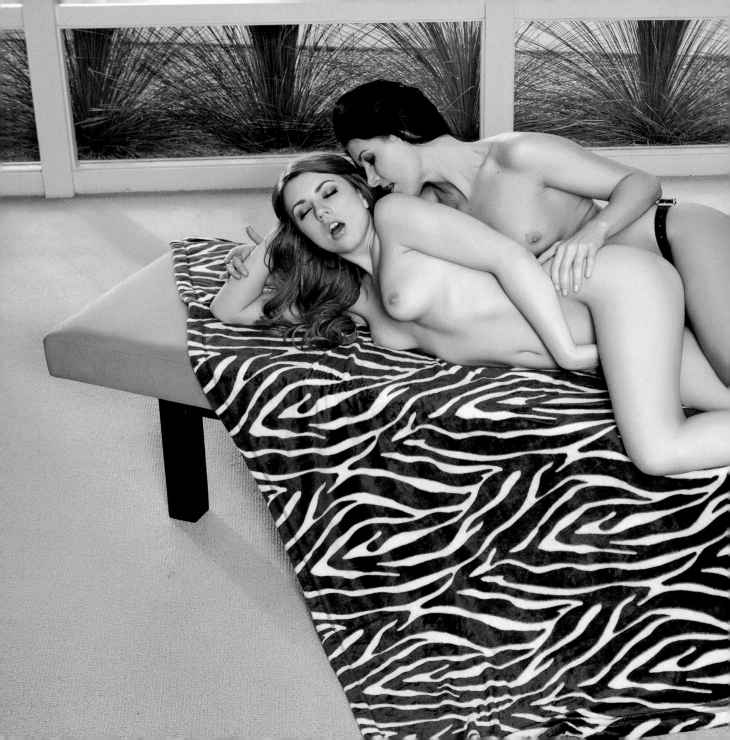

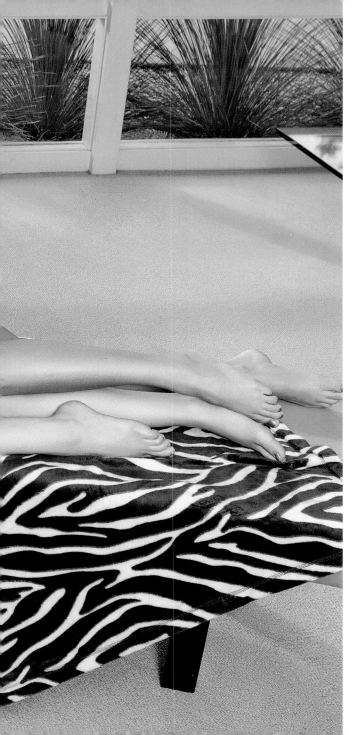

SPOON

Because Spoon facilitates shallower penetration, the head of his penis comes into contact with the G-spot with each stroke. It works well if you like a rear-entry position, but don't want deep or powerful thrusting. This position gives you a lot of skin-to-skin contact and closeness, although no face-to-face communication or eye contact.

1. Lie on your side with your partner lying behind you, curled against you so you fit together like two spoons in a tray.

2. He enters you from behind.

3. The same holds true for sex with a strap-on dildo, and a dildo with a pronounced or curved head works best.

4. Take Spoon to new heights: Ask your partner to reach around and stimulate your clitoris, or you can touch yourself.

COWGIRL

In the Cowgirl position, your partner lies on his back with his legs together, while you sit on top, straddling and facing him. Being on top puts you in the driver's seat: You take control of the angle, depth, and rhythm of penetration. You can tilt your body or rock your hips to find the perfect position to stimulate your G-spot.

1. Begin by sitting up straight, so your upper body forms a 90-degree angle with your partner's body.

2. Experiment with subtle changes in angle. Try leaning back and pushing your hips forward. Not only does your partner have a wonderful view of your body and the penetration action, but he also has easy access to your clitoris.

3. Next, lean forward, tipping your hips slightly downward.

4. Lean forward farther so you're almost lying on his chest.

5. Have him press his penis just above the pubic mound as you ride him, in order to increase the pressure on your G-spot.

6. People who are new to wearing a strap-on may want to try this position first, so your partner can do a lot of the work.

7. To bring some spice to Cowgirl, get up on your feet for more leverage and movement.

8. You can also switch directions and face away from your partner in Reverse Cowgirl. Depending on the curve of the penis or dildo, Reverse Cowgirl may feel better than Cowgirl, or vice versa.

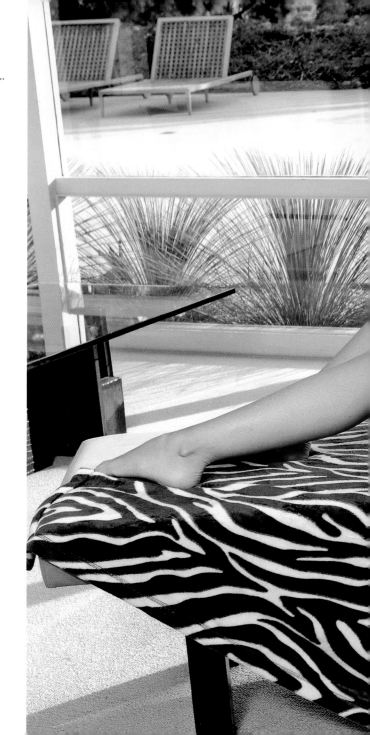

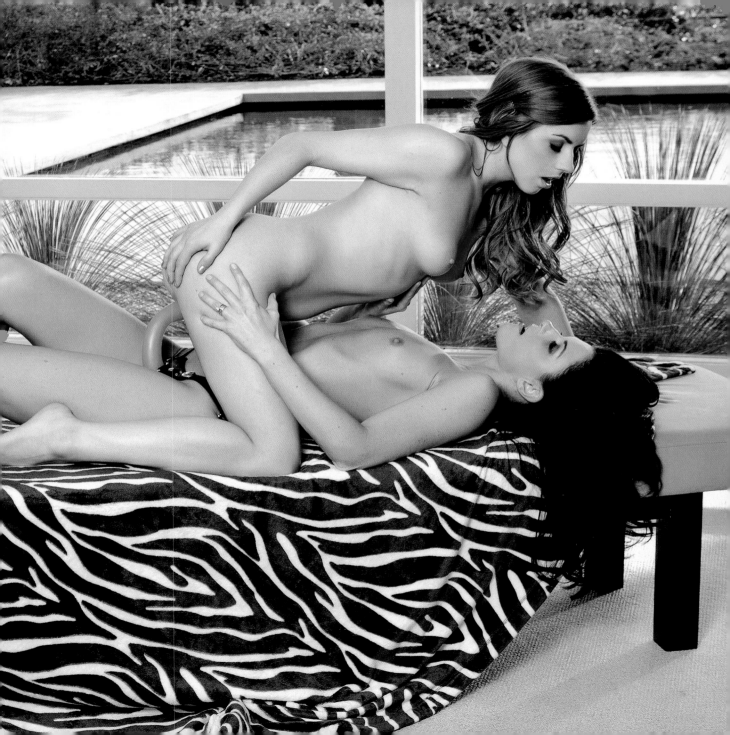

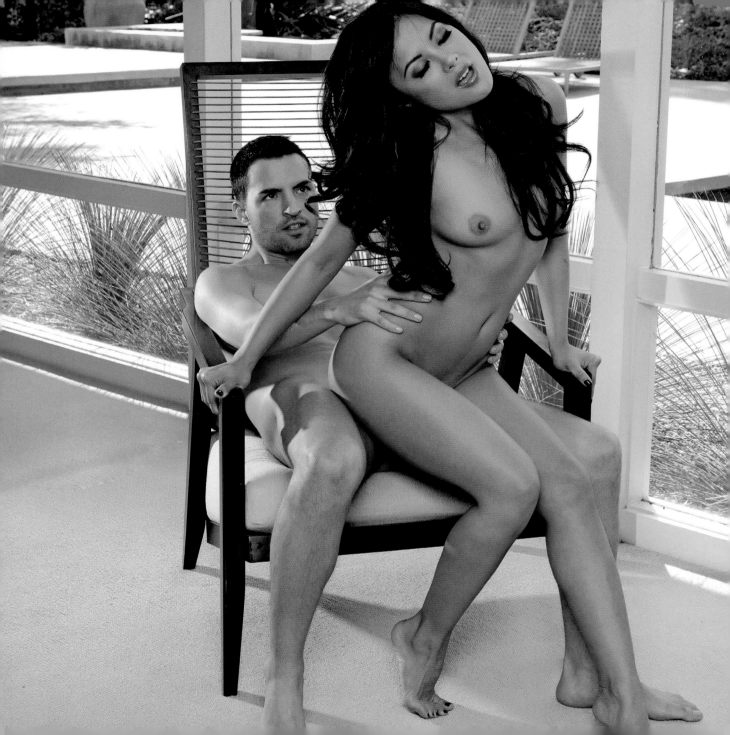

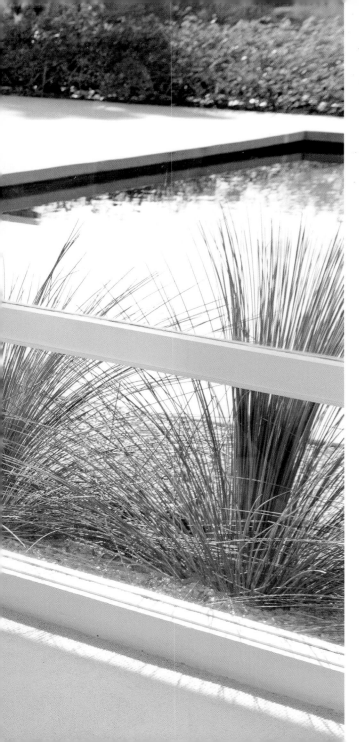

REVERSE CHAIRMAN

In Chairman position, your partner sits on a comfortable chair and you sit in his lap facing him, with your legs wrapped around him. Because he's sitting, he has less mobility and can take shorter strokes than in a position such as Doggie Style, and thereby hit your G-spot with each stroke.

1. In a variation called Reverse Chairman, you flip around so that you're sitting in his lap facing away from him with your legs together and your feet on the floor. If the chair has arms, you can use them for leverage; otherwise, put something in front of you to brace yourself.

2. He enters you from behind in this position.

3. You can adjust your body position by leaning back against him or leaning forward. If you're flexible enough, you may even be able to bend over and touch the floor.

4. Add the wow factor to Reverse Chairman by giving him (or her) a sexy lap dance first.

STRAP-ON TUTORIAL

To put on a harness, first buckle all the straps together, keeping it loose. Slip the dildo through the O-ring, and step into the harness as if it were a pair of underpants or shorts. Then position the dildo, adjust the straps, and tighten them. Or you can put the strap around your hips, slide the dildo through the O-ring, then buckle or fasten the other strap (or straps). Be sure to buckle or fasten the harness so it's tight against your body. A common mistake beginners make is leaving it too loose.

Position the dildo where it's most comfortable for you. Most people like it to sit against the pubic mound, so that the bottom of the dildo base rests against the clitoral hood and top of the vulva. If the dildo has a very exaggerated curve, make sure the curve is always aimed toward the front of your partner's body for G-spot stimulation.

Penetrating someone while wearing a strap-on is a learned skill, so give yourself some time to get the hang of it. As a woman doing the penetration, you should experiment with different positions. The first few times I did it, I had my partner in Doggie-Style position.

- This position allows for a good angle of penetration, toward the G-spot.

- The angle lets you keep your balance, establish a rhythm, and get some good thrusting going.

You may want to start out that way, but you can also try Missionary or Cowgirl.

Learning how to skillfully wield a strap-on takes practice and patience. If you feel like the dildo is moving around too much or it doesn't feel secure, then your harness isn't tight enough and you should adjust it. In the beginning, you may want to guide the dildo with your hand, which will give you more control of exactly where it's going.

1. When your partner is ready for penetration, be gentle and go slowly.

2. Press the tip of the well-lubricated dildo against her opening, and have her back onto it. This may help her feel less vulnerable, and will reassure you that you're not hurting her.

3. Once you are inside her, and she's ready for some movement, begin slowly.

4. You want to establish a thrusting motion with your hips, one that feels good to her and won't tire you out too quickly.

Wearing a strap-on enables women to experience many different levels of sexual enjoyment, emotionally and physically. The trust and intimacy between partners can feel especially heightened and very arousing. The naughty, taboo aspect of a woman with a dick can really get her motor going. The power she feels as the penetrating partner can add to her fantasy and pleasure. Strap-on sex also has the potential to be physically stimulating for the one wearing the dildo. For some women, the base of the dildo rubbing against the clitoris and vagina can create enough friction to feel fantastic. You can also choose a vibrating dildo, a harness with a pocket for a vibrator, or a double-ended dildo designed for use in a harness. With a double-ended dildo, one end slides inside the person wearing the harness and the other end extends out through the O-ring on the harness.

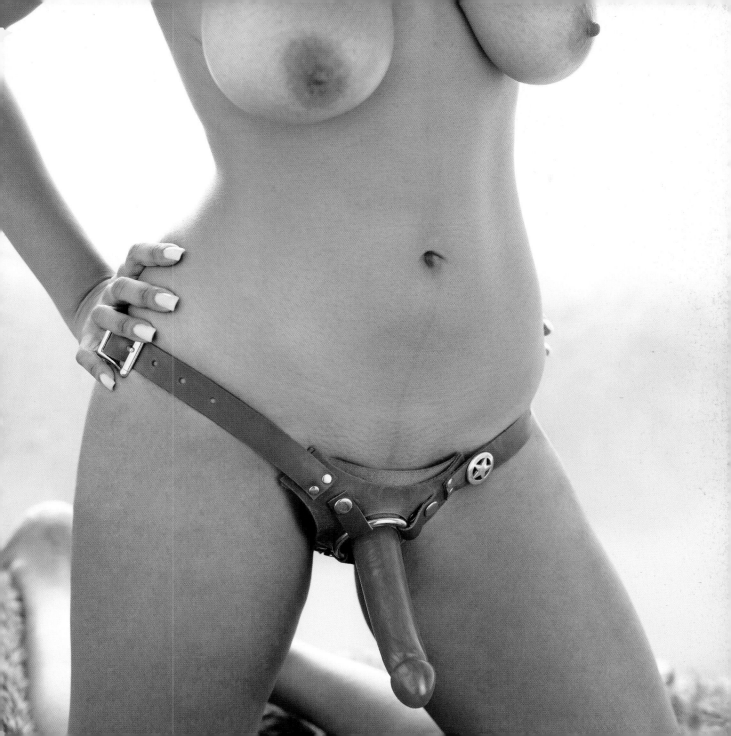

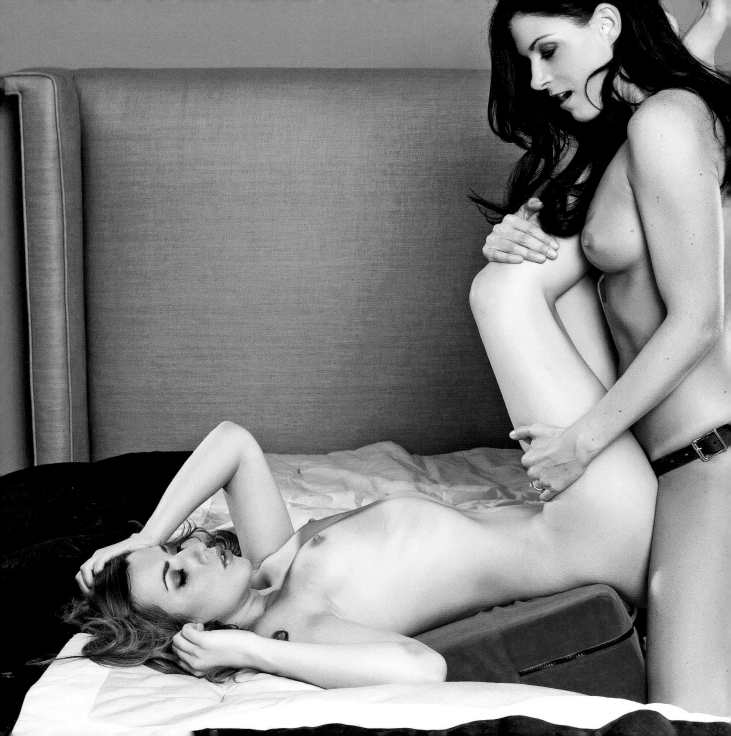

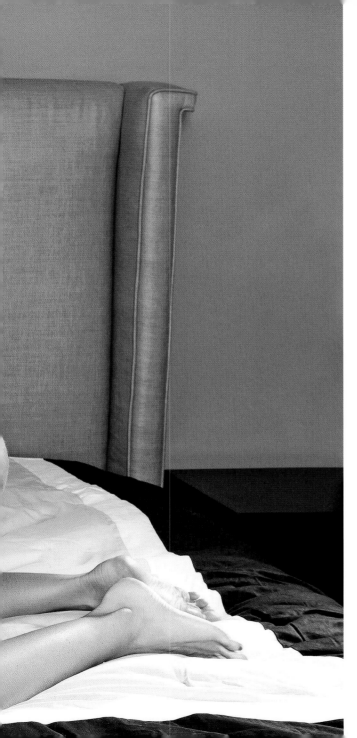

INVERTED SPIDER

In the Inverted Spider position, your pelvis is tipped upward, making it easier for him to slide against the G-spot as he penetrates you.

1. Lie on your back while your partner kneels between your legs.

2. Slowly raise your legs as your partner pulls your ankles toward his shoulders.

3. Lift your butt up and off the bed, so that you're supporting your weight on your upper back and shoulders.

4. Make Inverted Spider even more enjoyable (and more comfortable) with a Liberator Shape.

⌐ TRISTAN'S TIPS

Liberator Shapes are extra-firm pillows in different shapes that were designed especially for sex. They have soft, velvety covers that are removable, water resistant, and machine washable. They're great for people of all sizes and shapes, as well as those with back pain and other mobility issues. You can use the Liberator Wedge or Ramp underneath your body to achieve Inverted Spider position, get a good angle for G-spot stimulation, and get some support under your body.

MISSIONARY FOLD

If you like having sex on your back, know that it's not necessarily the ideal position for your G-spot. Try a variation of traditional Missionary position called Missionary Fold.

1. Lie on your back, bend your knees, and bring them up to your chest while your partner lies on top of you. This position curves his pelvis away from you slightly, allowing for a different angle of entry.

2. Depending on the curve of the penis or dildo, if your partner takes short strokes, there will be pressure on your G-spot.

3. If you're super flexible, you can fold your body in half and let your legs rest on your shoulders.

4. If you're using a strap-on, a curved dildo designed for the G-spot works fantastically in this position.

5. Add a little kink to Missionary Fold: Let your partner tie your wrists to the bedposts with silk scarves, or use bondage cuffs.

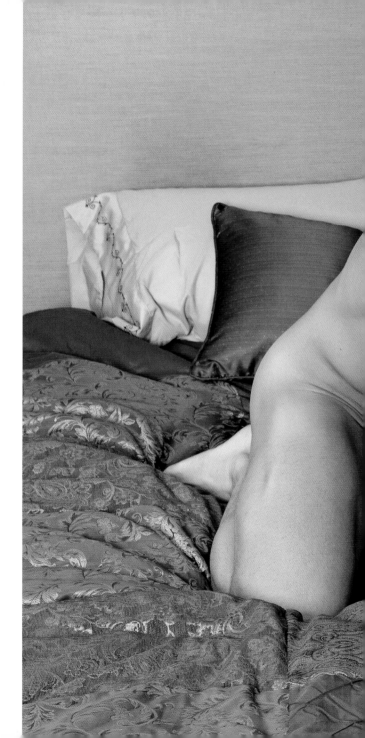

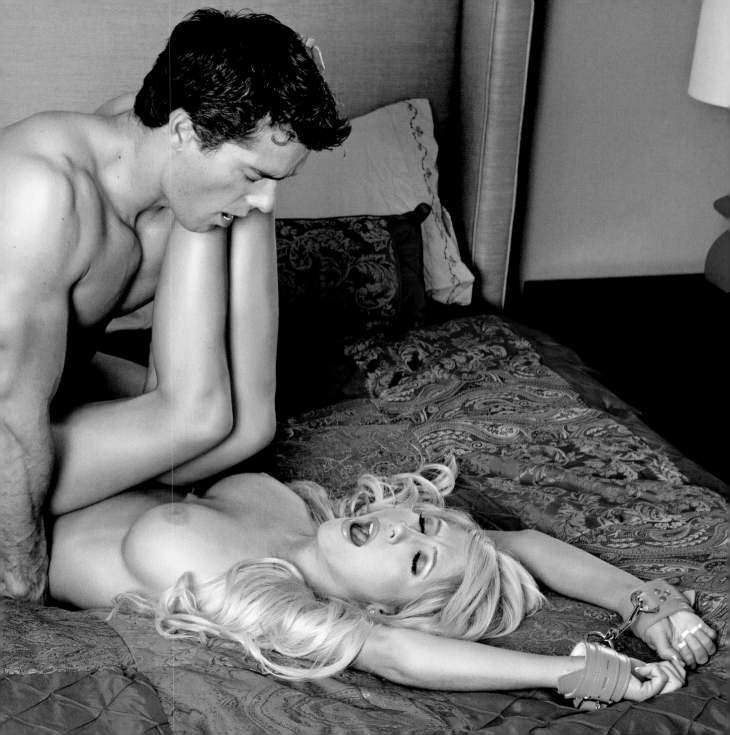

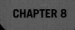

CHAPTER 8

FROM A TO G: ANAL PENETRATION AND G-SPOT STIMULATION

*When my ass is penetrated, I'm flooded with extreme physical sensations.
It's as if my entire genital region is electric and you just plugged me in.
The more turned on I get, the more I feel like my G-spot just comes alive.*

—Christie

You know you can stimulate the urethral sponge through the front wall of the vagina, but what has the ass got to do with the G-spot? Well, first let's recognize the merits of the ass on its own. It's an incredible erogenous zone rich in nerve endings. It's sensitive to stimulation, vibration, and penetration. It's a site of pleasure for many women. And one of the ways that women experience pleasure—and reach orgasm—from anal penetration is through indirect stimulation of the G-spot.

The first ingredient for great anal sex is desire. You've got to want anal sex wholeheartedly or it's just not going to work. If you feel nervous or pressured, your body will echo your ambivalence. Your sphincter muscles won't relax, your anus won't open up, and anal stimulation won't feel good. You've got to want it! You've also got to talk about it. Talk to your partner before anything happens, set the ground rules, and discuss any anxiety either of you may have. Keep up the communication during the experience. As the receiver, take the lead and let your partner know how everything feels and what you want.

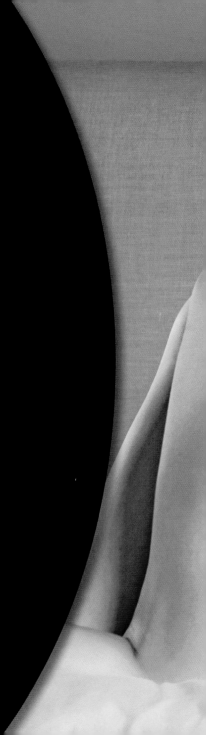

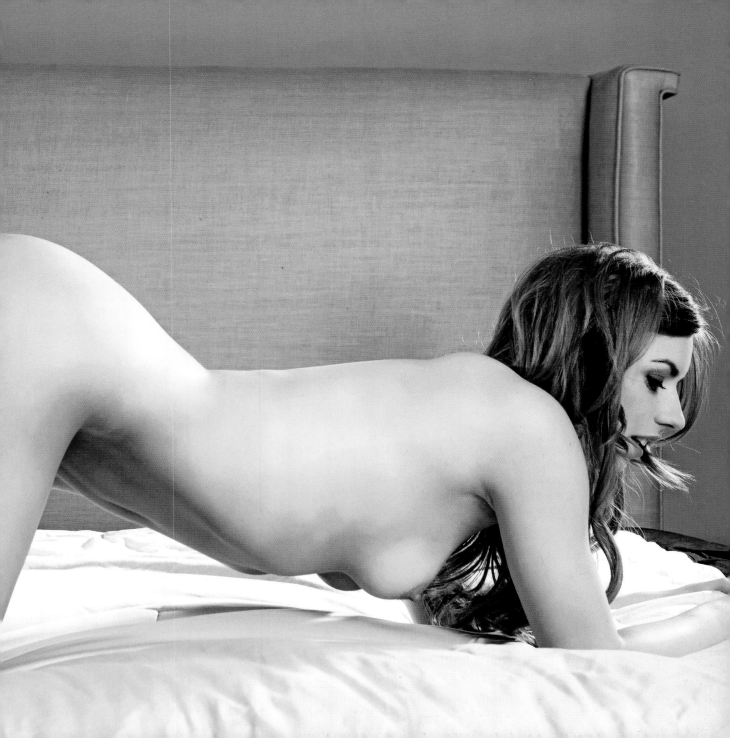

The rectum is not a straight tube, but has two gentle curves. The lower part of the rectum curves toward your navel. After a few inches, the rectum curves back toward your spine, then toward your navel again. The rectum and colon both curve laterally (from side to side) as well; whether they curve to the right or the left will vary from person to person. These curves are part of the reason that anal penetration should be slow and gentle, especially at first. Each person's rectum and its curves are unique, and it is best to feel your way into the rectum slowly, following its curves, rather than jamming something straight inside.

The anus, the anal canal, and the rectum are all sensitive in different ways, which is why anal stimulation and penetration can be so pleasurable. The anus and the outer part of the anal canal are made of the same sensitive soft tissue, and this tissue contains the greatest concentration of nerve endings of all our anal anatomy. In general, this tissue tends to be more sensitive to touch and vibration than the rectum. The inner part of the anal canal and the rectum are made of mucous membrane and have a lot fewer nerve endings; however, this tissue is much more sensitive to pressure (from penetration, for example).

A thin membrane separates the vaginal and rectal cavities. Many women can feel the sensitive area of the front wall of the vagina being stimulated through that membrane. Because of the curve of the rectum, you can experience pressure on the G-spot, especially in certain positions where your body is angled and with certain techniques that target the G-spot. Although that pressure may be less direct than during vaginal penetration, women say they can feel it intensely when they're having anal sex.

For some, this indirect stimulation of the G-spot—either in conjunction with clitoral stimulation or without it—is enough to bring them to orgasm. Others prefer a combination of vaginal and anal penetration for a double dose of G-spot stimulation. When something penetrates your rectum, your vaginal cavity narrows. So, with a dildo or penis in your ass and a finger or slim dildo inside your vagina, you could be on your way to G-spot ecstasy! Before you get there, let's go over the basics of anal sex and the best positions to help you hit the spot.

ANAL PENETRATION PRIMER

The ass is not self-lubricating, so you absolutely need to use lube, and plenty of it. You can use either water-based or silicone lube (as discussed in chapter 4), but stay away from numbing lubes. Some people prefer a thicker, water-based lube that is similar to the consistency of hair gel.

The key to safe, pleasurable anal sex is to slowly and patiently work your way up to intercourse. The biggest mistake people make is rushing the process, which leads to pain and frustration.

1. Start with plenty of warm-up, such as analingus and penetration with fingers, a butt plug, or a dildo. (Butt plugs are designed especially for anal play. They are intended to go in your ass and stay there during sex. Common styles have a teardrop shape, multiple beads, or a thick mushroom-cap head. They have a very slim neck underneath for the sphincter to close around, and a flared base at the bottom.)

2. If you're using fingers, make sure you have clean, well-filed short nails; you don't want to scratch the delicate tissue of the rectum. You can also slip on a latex or nitrile glove if you're practicing safer sex or you want to guarantee your fingers are butt-friendly.

3. If you use a toy, make sure the toy has a handle (for instance, at the end of a string of anal beads) or a flared base. Toys without a base or handle can get sucked into your rectum and stuck there. Let's avoid a trip to the emergency room, shall we?

4. Once a finger, toy, or penis has been in a woman's ass, don't put it in her vagina. Never go directly from ass to vagina because it can cause a vaginal infection. Either wash it or put a new glove or condom on it.

5. When you're playing with a woman's ass, don't neglect her clitoris. For some women, without clitoral stimulation, anal sex is not pleasurable; unless you attend to their clits, anal stimulation doesn't feel good. For others, adding clitoral stimulation—with oral sex, a hand, or a vibrator—intensifies the sensations of anal penetration and makes them better. Ask your partner about this; she may also want external stimulation of her vulva or vaginal penetration at the same time as anal penetration.

6. Anal sex should not hurt. If it hurts, you're not doing it right. If you start to feel any pain during penetration, don't panic—that will only make it worse. Take a deep breath, then another one. Sometimes, the initial penetration produces quite an intense feeling and you just need to relax, breathe deeply, and let your body get used to it.

7. If you do that and you're still feeling pain, have your partner slow down or pull out slightly, and see if that makes a difference. He may have to stop moving altogether; if he can do it and maintain his erection, have him simply stay inside you with little or no movement.

8. Add some more lube—too much friction may be causing the pain. Have him come out and switch back to whatever he was doing before the intercourse: two fingers, a butt plug, whatever it was. If none of these work and it still hurts, then stop altogether. It's crucial that you listen to your body.

PREPARATORY CLEANSING WITH AN ENEMA

Many people fear that anal sex is going to be dirty. Make sure you have a bowel movement as well as a bath or shower before you start exploring anal pleasure. Although it's not necessary, some people like to have an enema beforehand. An enema can loosen fecal matter, stimulate bowel movements, and clean out the anal canal and rectum. The simplest kind of enema is a disposable plastic bottle (found at drugstores) or a reusable rubber bulb syringe enema (available at sex and fetish stores). If you buy the drugstore kind, though, I recommend you dump out the liquid that comes in it, rinse out the bottle several times, then refill it with plain warm water. All store-bought enemas (including Fleet and other brands) contain a laxative. You don't need a laxative; you just need plain warm water.

To administer the enema, find a comfortable position. Some people like to lie on their sides, others like to squat over the toilet, others like to get in Doggie-Style position. Squeeze the water into your ass, hold the water until your body tells you it's time to go, and then have a bowel movement. Or you can fill the bottle, empty it into your ass, refill it, empty it into your butt again, then hold it for a few minutes until you feel the urge to go. Repeat the process until all that comes out of your ass is plain water.

You can also use an enema bag system. This requires the bag, tubing, a clamp, and a nozzle (sometimes sold all together in a kit at the drugstore), and is a little more complicated. Follow the instructions for use that come with the product. Because the bag holds up to 2 quarts (2 L) of water, some people say they get a deeper cleaning with an enema bag. It's your choice. Allow at least two hours between the end of your enema and the start of anal play. This gives your body a chance to recover and gives you time to make sure you're all cleaned out.

FOR NERVOUS BEGINNERS

If you are new to anal pleasure and nervous about it, before you explore it with your partner, try it with yourself. The next time you masturbate, incorporate some anal play into the mix. When you are by yourself, you can set the pace, go as slowly as you need to, and stop whenever you want. Because you're alone, the pressure of pleasing your partner is off the table and you can really concentrate on how you feel and what you want.

Solo sessions, during which you experiment with different toys and sensations, may help you find what works best for you and acquaint you with your ass in a new way. Begin with external stimulation until you're ready to move on to having something inside. You may choose to use your own fingers or a sex toy. Use plenty of lube and find a position that makes it easy for you to reach your anus. When you feel comfortable, you're ready to share the activity with your partner. All of your experimentation should come in handy, because you'll know more about what you like and what turns you on.

ANAL PLAY WITH FINGERS AND TOYS

I'll say it again: Fingers and toys aren't just for foreplay or warm-up. You can apply many of the same manual techniques described in chapter 6 for vaginal G-spot stimulation to the butt to achieve indirect G-spot stimulation. Remember to take it slow.

DIGITAL TECHNIQUE

1. To begin, your partner should lube his index finger and touch the pad of it to your anus.

2. Wait for the opening to relax, then he can slip his finger inside just to the first knuckle and stay there. Let your ass get used to the feeling of the finger. He should not make any sudden movements or try to go farther.

3. When the sphincter muscles begin to relax, he can venture farther inside.

4. Give your partner plenty of feedback about how all this feels. When you're ready for more, he can experiment with different sensations.

5. When his fingers are inside your ass, as with vaginal penetration, he should aim toward the front of your body.

6. He can use the classic "come here" technique with two hooked fingers or experiment with shorter, swifter movement and more pressure with his fingers.

7. Try a finger (or two) in your vagina and ass at the same time, moving them in concert to stimulate that sensitive spot on the front wall.

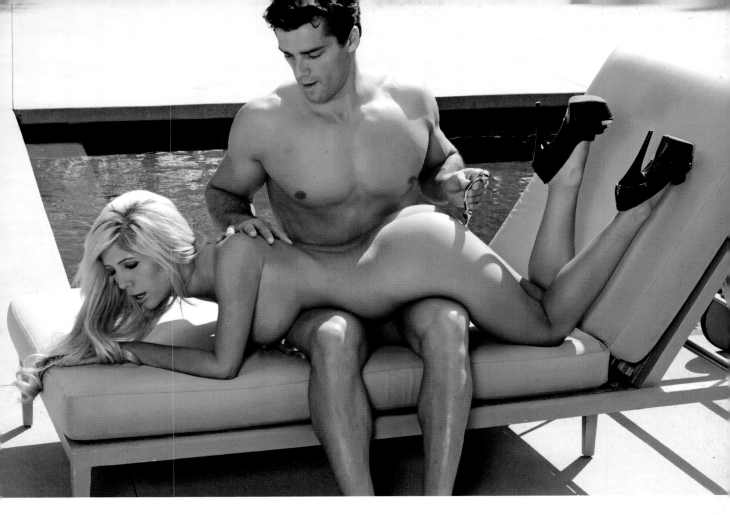

USING TOYS FOR ANAL PENETRATION

All of the G-spot dildos and wands already discussed also work well for anal penetration to give you indirect G-spot stimulation. As long as the toy has a base or a handle, it's safe to put in your ass. Remember to use plenty of lube and never go directly from ass to vagina. Keep in mind that the rectum is not a straight tube like the vagina; it has two gentle curves in it. So, a toy with a dramatic curve may feel better in one orifice than in the other.

TRISTAN'S TIPS

The Fun Wand by Njoy is a stainless steel S-shaped wand that's half the thickness of the Pure Wand discussed in chapter 6. One end is smooth with a single ball; the other end has three teardrop-shaped balls. Both ends are great for anal penetration—and the curve of the toy plus the solid texture of the metal ensure good indirect G-spot stimulation. Aim the curve toward the front of her body and use a pulling motion.

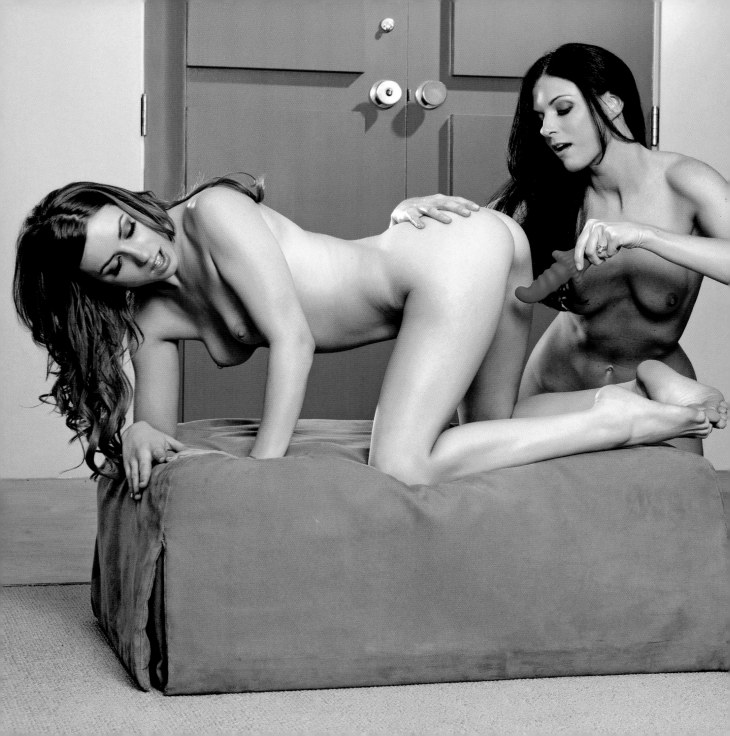

For anal play, the G-Swirl by Good Vibrations is a better choice than the vibrators discussed in chapters 3 and 4. It is a silicone insertable vibrator shaped like a hooked finger. Halfway down the shaft is a wider ring (which kind of resembles two wings). The shape of this vibrator makes it safe for anal penetration because the wings act as a base; when inserted into the rectum, they vibrate against the perineum and the anal opening. (When inserted vaginally, the wings vibrate against the clitoris and the perineum.) The vibration itself may provide enough indirect G-spot stimulation for you; if not, move the toy slowly in and out.

BEST POSITIONS FOR G-SPOT STIMULATION

It's a good idea to experiment with different positions, because G-spot stimulation has a lot to do with the angle of your body. Each position has its own pros and cons: how comfortable and sustainable it is, the level of face-to-face and/or skin-to-skin contact it affords, the depth and angle of penetration it creates, and the amount of thrusting and pressure it allows. You want to find a few positions that do the following:

1. Angle your body so that the penis or dildo can have as much contact as possible with the front wall of your vagina. Positions where your partner enters you from behind and slightly above achieve this nicely, as do positions where you are on top.

2. Give your partner the chance to do some powerful thrusting, to create firm pressure on the G-spot.

3. Create an angle of entry that lets the head of the penis or dildo hit the front wall just inside the vagina, rather than aiming toward the back of the vagina and the cervix.

SPOON

Spooning is a great position for beginners because your partner won't be able to thrust too vigorously or too deeply. Shallow, less powerful strokes are a good way for you to explore anal penetration without doing too much too soon.

Experiment with variations of your body position until you find just the right angle for indirect G-spot stimulation. For example, rather than keeping your legs together, you can swing one leg over your partner's top leg to change the angle of penetration. Bend your knees to give him easier access. Or you can move your upper body so you are leaning away from him.

You can easily stimulate your vulva and clitoris during penetration as well. This is a comfortable rear-entry position for lots of folks, regardless of body size or the size difference between their bodies. You don't have face-to-face communication, but you can turn your heads to kiss and sometimes look at each other.

DOGGIE STYLE

When people think of anal sex, Doggie Style is usually the first position that comes to mind. As with vaginal intercourse, when you put your head and shoulders down, your body is at a perfect angle for him to hit the G-spot. When he penetrates your ass in this position, his penis is at a sharper angle downward than when he penetrates your vagina, so pressure on the G-spot is easy to achieve. With you on your hands and knees and your partner behind you, he can see what he's doing (hey, those two holes are close together) and establish a good rhythm. You can stimulate your clitoris with your hand or a vibrator without it getting in the way.

This position can convert to Reverse Cowgirl when you're ready to get on top. If your bodies line up well, you can also try Stallion, where you're both standing (with you leaning against the bed and him behind you), and he may have better leverage that way.

HORIZONTAL TAILGATE

This is one of my favorite positions for both vaginal and anal intercourse. Like other rear-entry positions, in this one his penis is naturally aimed toward the front wall of your vagina. In the Tailgate position, you lie flat on your stomach with your legs spread slightly. Your partner sits on top of you with his legs on either side of yours and enters you from behind. To make it Horizontal Tailgate, once he penetrates you, he leans forward so he's lying on top of you. You can also begin in Doggie Style or Spoon position and transition to this position easily.

Many women like to feel the weight of a partner on top of them, which also adds to the pressure against your G-spot. Horizontal Tailgate may not be feasible if your partner is a lot bigger than you and you can't support his or her weight. Regardless of your partner's size, some women may feel too confined or uncomfortably pinned down.

MISSIONARY L

This is a very good position for women who like direct and indirect G-spot stimulation at the same time. However, this variation of Missionary position can be difficult to sustain for women with limited flexibility or mobility—if that describes you, try this one, with caution.

1. While you lie on your back, he kneels between your legs and sits on the backs of his calves.

2. Extend your legs straight up in front of him so that they are perpendicular to the rest of your body (your body forms an "L" shape). Holding your legs at a right angle to your torso straightens out the rectum slightly and makes anal penetration a little easier.

3. He can slide a hand between your legs and press above your pubic mound, creating external pressure on the G-spot.

4. He can slip a well-lubed finger or a slim dildo or vibrator inside your vagina and make a "come here" motion toward himself.

5. Or, if he's busy working on your ass, you can grab the toy yourself and take care of the front while he takes care of the back.

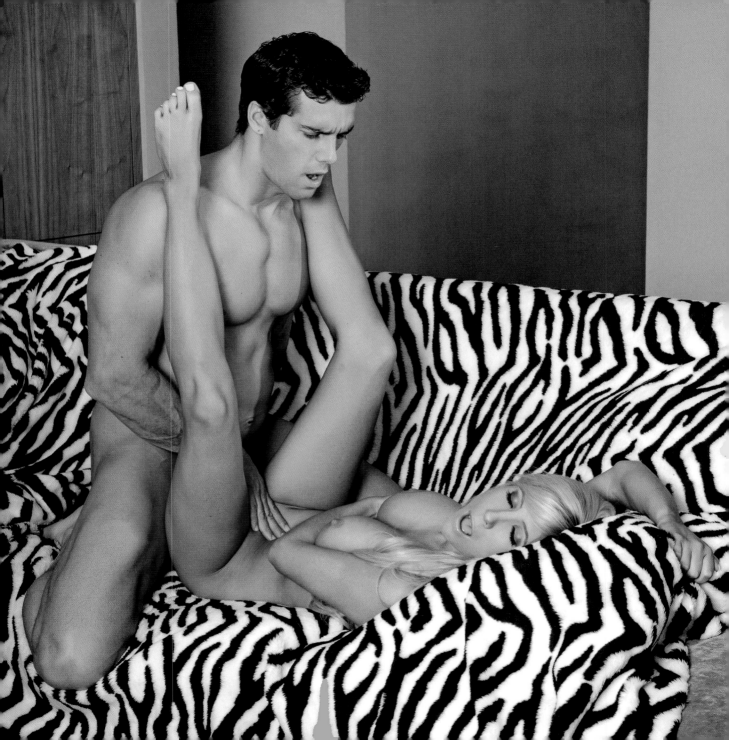

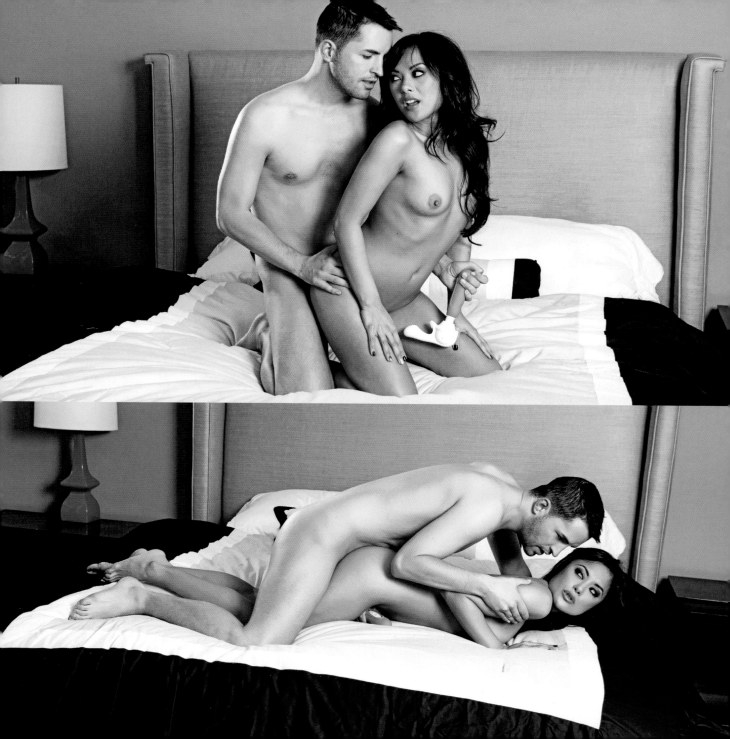

GREAT TOY/POSITION COMBO: HORIZONTAL TAILGATE + MYSTIC WAND + G-SPOT ATTACHMENT

talked about the Hitachi Magic Wand in chapter 3, but there's another wand that will really drive you wild: the Mystic Wand by Vibratex. Because it's more compact than the Magic Wand (although some folks say not quite as powerful), it is easy to use for clitoral stimulation during anal intercourse with a partner. It's also cordless and rechargeable, so no plug or extension cord is necessary—and it's made of silicone, so it's easy to clean. Beyond being a great clitoral vibrator, it can also be transformed into a G-spot toy with the G-spot Attachment. Like the Gee Whiz for the Magic Wand, this silicone attachment fits over the head of the Mystic Wand, making it insertable.

If you enjoy anal intercourse with clitoral stimulation, then I've got a setup for you. Get into Horizontal Tailgate position and slip the Mystic Wand underneath you. Slide the attachment inside your vagina until the textured nubby exterior sits comfortably against your clit and vulva. Have your partner enter your ass. The pressure of something in your ass, your partner's weight on you, and the insertable part of the vibrator in your vagina is a surefire combination for a rockin' orgasm!

REVERSE COWGIRL

To take charge of the penetration and set the pace and the rhythm, you want to be on top. This position offers you the flexibility to tweak the arc of your body to hit the G-spot and get it just right. In Reverse Cowgirl position, you straddle his body and face away from him. You can sit down on his penis, going as slowly as you need to, which gives him a great view of the penetration and your butt.

Take advantage of all your options: Lean forward or backward, shift your hips, and tilt your pelvis to come up with an angle that gives you the most pressure on your G-spot. It all depends on the curve of his penis, your internal shape, and how you line up with one another. If his penis has a significant curve toward him when it's erect, then facing each other in Cowgirl position may be better for G-spot stimulation.

EROTIC INTERLUDE #2: "GIRL TALK"

BY RACHEL KRAMER BUSSEL

My three best friends and I were gathered for our monthly Sunday brunch. We saw each other occasionally during the rest of the month, but this was our special, sacred time to dish—especially about sex.

"So, Tanya, what have you been up to? I know we've probably only heard a sliver of it," I teased her, trying to focus on my most glamorous friend, rather than on the afterglow I could still feel from the way Pete had worked his fingers inside me as a wake-up call this morning. I squirmed as she winked at me.

"Well, I had a foursome last night, with Billy, my latest boy toy, and a couple we met. We were up pretty much all night, culminating with them pouncing on me, all three of them. They even made me squirt!"

Whoa. I wasn't expecting her to steal my thunder like that, and apparently neither were Ellie and Juliet, because they leaned in excitedly.

"Tell us more!" Ellie squealed, sucking on the straw of her daiquiri almost violently.

I listened as Tanya regaled us with the story of how Billy had played with her nipples while the guy, Jake, had kissed her and Maya had started playing with her pussy. Just hearing about it made me tingle all over again. "And then she must've found my G-spot. No one had ever touched me like that. You know what that's like, right?"

Ellie and Juliet both shook their heads, but I smiled. "I know exactly," I said. I had to keep my normally loud voice low. "I just have to tell you about what Pete does to me. He has magic hands—magic, I tell you."

The waiter arrived and I ordered the first thing I saw on the menu, not really caring what I ate as long as I got to relive the way my man coaxed orgasm after orgasm out of me.

"Well, you know how I've always had trouble coming? I mean, I do, but it takes forever. But with Pete, I don't have that problem. In fact, he gets me so worked up it's like my G-spot wants to be found." I looked around, gauging their reactions, because a good sex story isn't just about whether you enjoyed it, but about making sure your friends enjoy it, too.

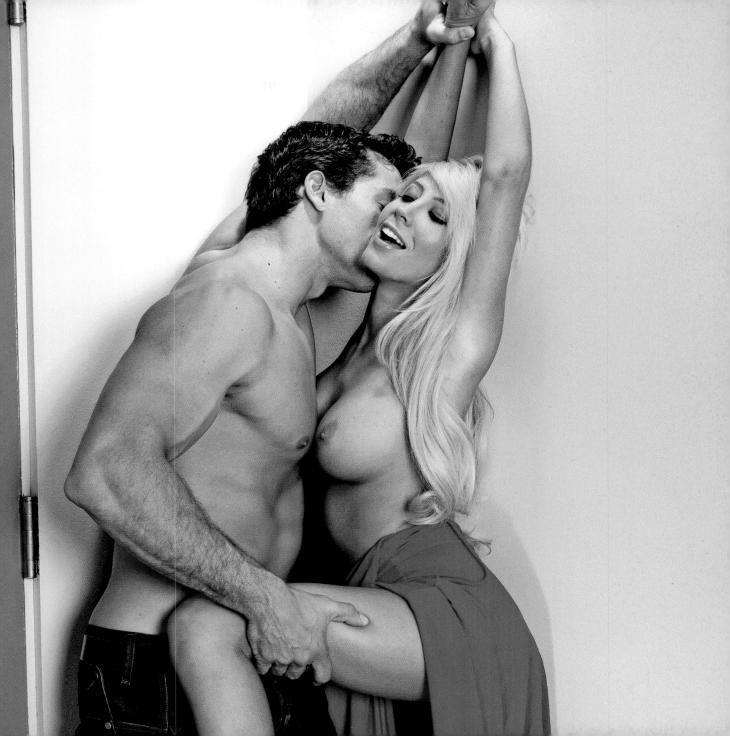

"He loves using his fingers on me—I mean loves it. I've never been with anyone who was so good at that, and who wanted to do it so often. I'll try to pause and do something for him but he likes to watch me, and he just manages to make me feel like I'm exploding."

They were all still looking at me, so I went on. "And it keeps going and going, like when I start to give him a blow job, he starts touching me, and not just a little bit, but really twisting his fingers inside me, until I almost can't concentrate on what I'm doing. He'll say, 'Keep going, Amy,' and I do, because how can I stop? He moves kind of slowly, not that pushing in and out a lot of guys try, like it's a mechanical exercise. He somehow gets his fingers into a part of me that makes it feel so good, and I just want to gush."

"Your G-spot," Tanya said knowingly.

"Exactly. But he teases me, and draws it out, and all of it makes me open wider and then finally when I think I can't stand it anymore, he tells me to hold still, with his dick between my lips, and makes me come all over his fingers. It's truly incredible."

I finished my sentenced and felt the heat upon my cheeks; even a girl as open as I am about sex can still get a little embarrassed. I let the other girls take over the conversation, suddenly craving Pete's fingers for dessert.

After brunch, I rushed home to find Pete in front of his computer, intent on some video game. I'd taken my panties off in the car and put them in my purse. A wet pussy is no match for even the most heated game, at least not with my guy.

He paused and looked up at me with a smile when I walked in, and my whole body tingled. He has a way of making even sitting still sexy; I've come to believe it's because he's able to put his whole focus on me, on us, when we're intimate. He doesn't want me to come because it'll make him look good, puff him up with pride, like some of my former lovers, but because it'll make me feel good, make me cry out, make me experience the ultimate pleasure.

"How was brunch?" he asked, his tone casual, though I sensed something hidden beneath his words.

"It was fun. I told them all about what you do to me."

"Everything?" he asked as I approached, straddling his lap and letting his wandering hand discover when it hit my bare ass that I was pantyless.

"Pretty much. They wanted to know your secrets."

"I don't have any, I don't think, but I do have a surprise," he said, grinning mischievously.

"For me?" I asked.

He knows I love presents, no matter how small. I live for the unexpected, which is perhaps why his ability to make me come and come and come, keep my pussy wet and my mind aroused, was such a shock to my way of life at age thirty-five. I hadn't expected a lover to come along and truly rock my world, but he had done that and then some.

"Yes, for you, but first you have to do something for me."

"Anything," I said, smiling as I leaned in for a kiss.

He granted me the kiss, his tongue sliding easily into mine. He tasted like smoke, and even though I hate the fact that he smokes, I love the taste of him no matter what. I reached up to stroke his stubble, but he pushed my hand away.

"Wait," he said. "Close your eyes and hold out your hands."

I did, immediately, eager to see what he'd gotten me. Less than a minute later he was back, placing something solid and cool against my hands.

"What is it?" I asked, even though I could tell it was a vibrator. I own several, and enjoy them with and without Pete.

"It's a special toy, just for you. It's for your G-spot. I want to use it on you, and I want you to use it while I'm doing other things to you, and when I'm not here, so you can tell me about it."

In all the years I'd been using vibrators, no one had ever bought me one as a gift, and certainly no lover had ever been as thoughtful. Pete had selected a toy in my favorite color: purple. Just holding it in my hand made me feel giddy.

Part of me wanted to protest, though; after all, we had his hands, his magic, heat-seeking hands, the ones that seemed designed to press against exactly the parts of me I needed him to. Pete knows when to go deeper, when to add more fingers, and when a gentle touch is all I need to get off. But I kept quiet, because I didn't want to insult him, and I was thrilled that he'd been thinking about more ways to please me.

"Just so you know, you weren't the only one talking about our sex life. I described you to the salesgirl where I bought this. I could've bought it online, but I wanted to hold them and get an expert opinion. I told her how wet you get, how responsive you are, how your G-spot is already getting a workout, but that I wanted you to feel something bigger and better. This was the one she recommended."

I blushed thinking about him sharing those details; it was one thing for me to freely share details about him, but another for him to talk about me. I liked it, though, and I especially liked that he went to so much trouble to find something I'd appreciate.

"You're wearing too many clothes," he said, smiling at me not just with his beautiful lips but also with his deep brown eyes.

"Is this better?" I asked, lifting my leopard-print dress over my head and kicking off my boots. My breasts are just big enough that I should wear a bra, but sometimes I leave them bare, and today I was grateful for leaving them free. My hard nipples popped out toward him, and he pulled me close, grabbing my ass with one hand and sucking a nipple into his mouth with the other. Immediately, I felt an intense tugging

deep inside. It was almost painful, but I knew that soon he'd fill me and, in doing so, give me what my pussy was searching for as it pulsed with need.

"Are you ready?" he whispered as he pulled away, and I nodded. He sank down to the ground and pulled my hips close, teasing the very edge of my sex with his tongue, then sucking on my clit for a few seconds before pressing inside.

"More," I couldn't help whispering as he ate me lustily.

He loves going down on me, and I love the feel of his warm tongue against me, but even more than that, I desire firm pressure, the feeling of pressure there, right there, where it feels like I will burst into pieces, so for us, oral sex is more of a form of teasing foreplay than anything else. He took the toy and rubbed its curved purple head against my opening, and I sank down just a little to urge it inward.

"Relax, baby," he said. "Easy does it."

And with that, he both pushed it inside and turned it on. I clutched for Pete's hair, gripping it firmly as the toy took me for a ride, like my own personal roller coaster, only this one was strictly for adults. He was sliding it gently in and out, then when it was deep inside, rocking it back and forth.

"That's it, Amy, keep going," he said, even though he was the one truly controlling the action. For him it was never about "giving" me an orgasm, but about me claiming what was rightfully mine as a woman.

"Aaah," I said, tears filling my eyes, happy tears, the kind that sometimes leak out when he's got three big fingers twisting inside me just right.

This toy was like that only more so, its vibrations strong and powerful. Standing made everything more intense, like I might collapse if I didn't hold on to him tightly. Slowly, I inched forward, so I could wrap my arms around Pete's head.

"Why don't we move over here?" he asked as he felt me shaking with my pending climax.

He eased the toy out, and I stared in fascination; it was covered with my juices.

"Lie down on your back," Pete said, and I did, spreading my legs wide. I'm never shy around him; he's brought out my exhibitionist side, and in fact I love showing off for him. So when he said, "Hold your legs up," I did, exposing everything down below. "Good girl."

He watched me for a few seconds, then ran his finger along my wetness again, even though I was clearly ready for much more than a lone finger. "What do you want, Amy?" he asked as he pressed the purple tip of the vibrator against me, letting me feel its possibilities but not sticking it in. I hate it when he teases me, but I also love it, too; he's so good at knowing when I'm ready to claw the sheets if I don't get well and truly fucked.

"I want you," I said, realizing as I did that even though the toy felt incredible, I wanted him—his fingers, his cock, his body on top of me.

"I'll give you everything you want, baby, but first we're going to make sure that clerk was right about this toy."

He pushed it inside again, and with my pussy so primed, and open, it seemed to zero right in on where I wanted it. I could just lie back and savor the feeling of it buzzing against my swollen insides, making me wetter and wetter.

"I like how wet it's making you, so wet for my cock," he said, lightly stroking my clit as the vibe went to town.

I bucked up against it, experimenting with tightening my walls around it, and as it turned out, everything I did felt amazing. Pete took his time, though the toy didn't; he revved it up to its maximum capacity, and it made me feel like I was spinning, rocketing up and up and up, somewhere far, far away, then pulled me right back into my center.

"That's it, honey, that's it," he said, and my orgasm felt like a jolt inside me.

I didn't make noise, like I usually do; I had my eyes scrunched tight. I didn't realize how much tension I'd been holding inside me until that orgasm wiped it all away, making me let loose in every sense of the word as the sexual fireworks went off inside me.

He pulled the toy out and climbed on top of me. "Are you ready, or do you want some time?"

Sometimes I have to wait after coming, to catch my breath and recover, but all I wanted was him. He slid his cock inside me, then positioned himself almost as if he were doing pushups, his arms on either side of me, his dick entering at an angle that ensured its head moved along all my most sensitive parts.

"Harder!" I exclaimed into his ear, but instead of giving me a proper pounding, he eased out and gave me just one strong thrust at a time, his eyes remaining on mine the whole time.

He wanted me to lose control, while he stayed calm and steady, even though I knew he was just as aroused as I was. That was what did me in, ultimately—well, that and the way each consecutive slam of his dick further engorged my insides. The toy had only been a teaser, a wonderful one, and now his cock was delivering on its promise. When he pressed his weight against me, crushing me beneath him and kissed the side of my neck, I pushed upward, intent on getting him all the way inside. But my Pete had other plans, as he often does, and instead of giving me more of his dick, he pulled out and pressed his fingers inside instead. I couldn't tell you how many—two, three, four?—but however many there were, they felt incredible. Blissful. Just beyond.

He curled them tight and wiggled them around and lifted his face to look at me so intently I couldn't look away. "I love how you feel like this, so raw, so open, so ready," he said, and then pulled out only to bring his cock back inside me.

He kept switching off and my inner walls seemed to tighten so much I was amazed he could fit himself inside me. But he did, again and again, until he finally gave in and gave me those hard, fast, solid thrusts, with my legs now propped up on his shoulders that signaled he was looking for a climax, too.

"You're so wet and tight," he murmured, as if to himself.

I focused on squeezing him, which wasn't hard after the sexual workout he'd just given me. When he grabbed my hands and pinned me down, so it felt as if the only part of me I could move was my pussy, I reveled in being his, fully, completely, forever his to enjoy and savor and surprise.

"Yes!" I screamed, or at least, that's what I tried to scream; what came out may have been more incoherent, because the noise that filled my head when I came, followed by him coming inside me, was so loud it took over everything else. I shuddered, clinging to him as long as I could.

"That's something new for you to talk about with the girls, isn't it?" he whispered in my ear.

I giggled, then hugged him tight. It certainly was.

RACHEL KRAMER BUSSEL (rachelkramerbussel.com) is a New York–based author, editor, and blogger. Her books include *Best Bondage Erotica 2011, Orgasmic, Fast Girls, Passion, The Mile High Club, Bottoms Up, Spanked, Peep Show, Tasting Him,* and more.

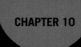

CHAPTER 10

G IS FOR GRATIFICATION: G-SPOT ORGASMS

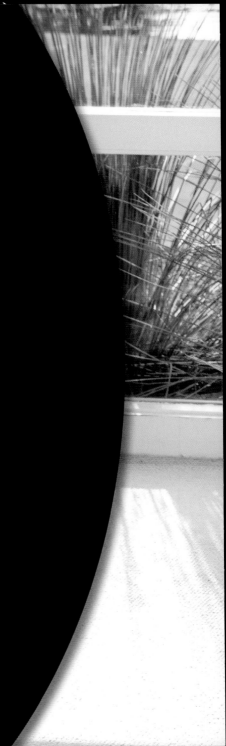

For me, a G-spot orgasm is more intimate than a clitoral orgasm. A clitoral orgasm starts outside my body, the stimulation is external, the sensations are primarily on the surface, and I can control how engaged I am in the encounter. A G-spot orgasm involves a different level of intimacy, because it's all inside. I have to surrender to the sensation and allow the other person inside deeply, and if I engage my breathing with the rest of the sensations: wow. A G-spot orgasm is not a release like a clitoral orgasm; it doesn't leave me feeling as though my physical body has shattered into millions of pieces. The G-spot orgasm is voluptuous and full and becomes more and more so, afterwards leaving me feeling powerful and sensual and like the most fuckable being that has ever existed. It's my favorite thing ever.

—Cat

Orgasms are like snowflakes—well, snowflakes that could shake the earth underneath you. They are individual, unique, and beautiful. Some orgasms are genitally focused, whereas others resonate from the tips of your toes to the top of your head, and plenty fall somewhere in between. Some orgasms are very quiet and internal, some are quick and explosive, others are intense and overwhelming, and others are wild and uninhibited.

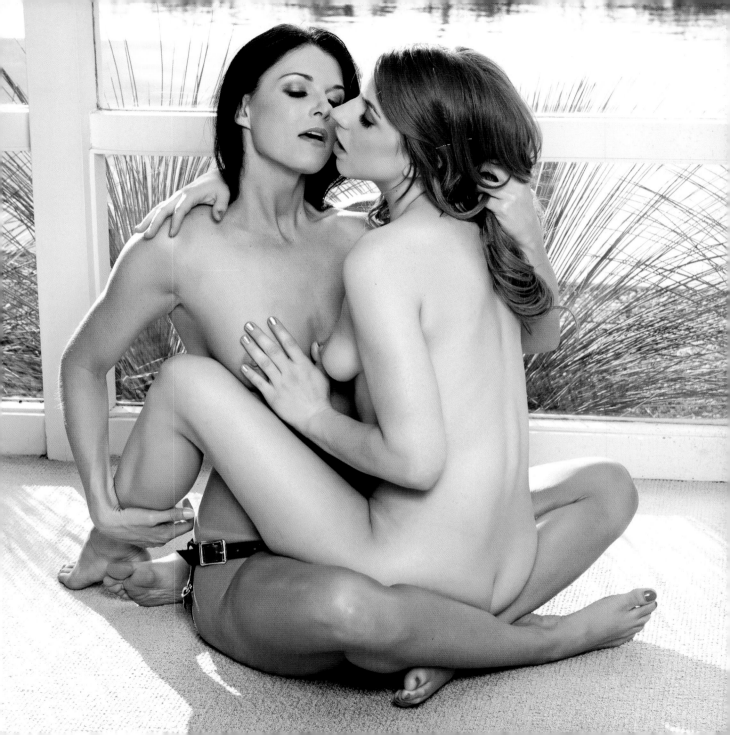

All women experience orgasm differently, but there are some commonalities in terms of physical changes. Muscle contractions occur in the uterus, vagina, and sphincter. Other muscles in the body contract as well, and you may experience muscle tension throughout your body—the entire body might tense or your hands and feet cramp at the peak of orgasm. Your body may spasm or tense up completely, then relax. You might make strange faces, or appear to be in pain or frowning, but it's actually an involuntary muscle response. Your skin flushes. Your heart can race and you may take shorter breaths. I've also seen women's pupils dilate, or their eyes appear to roll back into their heads. These are all signs that you're coming. Of course, you might also moan, scream, wail, or—partners appreciate this—announce it.

An orgasm can last anywhere from three seconds to several minutes. When you have an orgasm, lots of happy chemicals are released in your brain, including endorphins and naturally occurring steroids. What makes a G-spot orgasm different and sets it apart from other orgasms? To answer that question, we need a brief history lesson.

THE EVOLUTION OF THE FEMALE ORGASM

The female orgasm itself hasn't evolved dramatically. The science, research, and theories—our understanding of the female orgasm—are what have evolved. Ideas about the female orgasm are directly linked to those about female sexuality in general, and scientific, medical, and psychological theories about female sexuality have a pretty checkered past.

At the end of the nineteenth century, Sigmund Freud pronounced vaginal intercourse *the* way for women to experience pleasure and orgasm. According to Freud, women who got pleasure from clitoral stimulation were immature and stuck in adolescence. This idea was widely accepted, in the medical establishment and elsewhere, and women who weren't satisfied by intercourse were labeled frigid or even crazy. Freud's concept survived for fifty more years, into the twentieth century, until famed sexologist Alfred Kinsey turned everything upside down with his groundbreaking research.

In 1953, Kinsey released *Sexual Behavior in the Human Female* based on a study of nearly six thousand women, a huge sample compared with other research. In it, Kinsey proclaimed there was a single source for women's sexual response and pleasure: the clitoris. Therefore, all orgasms were clitoral orgasms. Sexologists and the general public enthusiastically adopted this idea, and it dominated our thinking about the female orgasm for decades. Although Kinsey's findings validated many women's experiences and empowered them to explore their sexual autonomy, those who experienced orgasm without clitoral stimulation were left pretty confused.

In their 1966 book *Human Sexual Response*, William H. Masters and Virginia E. Johnson didn't diverge far from Kinsey. They argued that although there can be different kinds of stimulation of different areas of the genitals that lead to orgasm, all orgasms are essentially the same. Their theory was based on their research, which found a similar physiological pattern among their subjects before, during, and after orgasm. This is the mapping of the female arousal cycle discussed in chapter 2, which includes four phases: excitement, plateau, orgasm, and resolution. Subsequently, other researchers challenged Masters and Johnson's findings about just how similar these physiological changes were, arguing instead that women's bodies behave differently depending on the kind of orgasm they are having.

Another school of thought began to emerge, and other sex researchers put forth a more complex explanation that included different types of female orgasms. Among them were Josephine and Irving Singer. In 1972, the Singers theorized that there were three different types of female orgasms: a vulval orgasm (achieved via clitoral stimulation), a uterine orgasm (which resulted from penetration and "cervical jostling"), and a blended orgasm, which had elements of both vulval and uterine orgasms. Penetration—and its orgasmic possibilities—finally came back into the picture.

DEFINING THE G-SPOT ORGASM

Women experience sexual desire, pleasure, and orgasm in myriad ways. Oral sex, penetration with fingers, intercourse, clitoral stimulation, vibrators, nipple stimulation, anal play, and fantasy can all be paths to orgasm. Researchers know—and I know from talking to thousands of women over the years—that many women have orgasms from G-spot stimulation alone or G-spot stimulation in combination with something else (such as clitoral stimulation).

CLITORAL, VAGINAL, AND UTERINE ORGASMS

The concept of a G-spot orgasm was first explored at the same time as the concept of the G-spot emerged—in the 1980 book *The G-Spot: And Other Discoveries About Human Sexuality*. In it, Alice Ladas, Beverly Whipple, and John Perry adapted the Singers' theory and put forth their own version of an orgasm continuum. It placed the clitoral orgasm at one end, the vaginal orgasm at the other end, and the blended orgasm in the middle of the continuum. They listed the G-spot as the main "trigger point" for a vaginal orgasm.

They argued that clitoral orgasms involved the pudendal nerve, a sensory, autonomic, and motor nerve that carries signals to and from the genitals, anal area, and urethra. Vaginal orgasms involved the pelvic nerve, which extends upward from the internal organs to the middle of the spinal cord and is believed to connect the G-spot to the spinal cord. Blended orgasms involved both. Ladas, Whipple, and Perry were the first researchers to propose that different nerve networks were involved in different types of orgasms. The authors' research subjects described clitoral orgasms as external and more localized to the genitals. They described blended and vaginal (G-spot) orgasms as more internal, deeper, and spread throughout the body. Ladas, Whipple, and Perry concluded that most women experience blended orgasms.

In her 2003 book *Female Ejaculation and the G-Spot*, Deborah Sundahl also takes the Singer model and creates a continuum similar to that of Ladas, Whipple, and Perry. At one end of her continuum is a clitoral orgasm, during which you experience rhythmic contractions of the PC muscles, you take short, quick breaths, and the orgasm feels insatiable.[9] A uterine orgasm is at the opposite end, and Sundahl (borrowing heavily from the Singers) describes it like this:

> Uterine orgasms are deeply emotional and satisfying and take place only if something, such as a penis, dildo, or fingers, is in contact with the cervix. Strong, deep, quick thrusting jostles the uterus . . . These orgasms do not

involve the rhythmic contractions of the PC muscles. Breathing is suspended (the apnea response) for 20 to 30 seconds just prior to climax.[10]

In the middle of Sundahl's continuum is a G-spot orgasm, which combines elements of orgasms from clitoral stimulation and deep penetration (with cervical contact): The G-spot orgasm produces PC muscle contractions and short breaths like a clitoral orgasm and has the emotional resonance and deep relaxing feeling of a uterine orgasm. Think of it as the best of both worlds.

Although plenty of sexologists and sex educators have classified orgasms in various ways, I want to acknowledge that categorization can be tricky territory. Although it may make sense for scientists to say "this is a clitoral orgasm," it may not be that simple for the woman having the orgasm. For example, clitoral stimulation techniques can vary: The orgasm you have from your own hand during masturbation can feel quite different from the orgasm you have when your partner goes down on you. Likewise, G-spot stimulation with a vibrator may lead to an orgasm that feels different than your orgasm from G-spot stimulation via vaginal penetration.

But we've got to start somewhere in order to talk about all this. So, I'm going to define a G-spot orgasm as an orgasm achieved primarily through G-spot stimulation. It does not have to, but may also include vulva, clitoral, and/or anal stimulation.

WHAT DOES A G-SPOT ORGASM FEEL LIKE?

What does a G-spot orgasm feel like? Based on both the research and women's descriptions, we can identify some basic elements:

- A G-spot orgasm feels less genitally focused than an orgasm from clitoral stimulation, and more like it is spreading throughout the body.

- Women often describe it as a deeper orgasm—they can feel contractions deep in the vaginal walls and even the uterus.

- Others say it lasts longer than other kinds of orgasms; it feels like a big release of tension, and/or it feels more intense.

- Deborah Sundahl makes the argument in her book that the G-spot "is a gateway to deeper aspects of sexual expression and intimacy."[11]

- Some say it feels more emotional; they may feel strongly connected to their bodies, their partners, or even the universe.

When asked to describe a G-spot orgasm, some women say it just feels *different*. That may sound vague, but considering all the different ways we can come, each orgasm *does* feel different. No orgasm is better or worse. Our orgasms produce different sensations and reactions, resonate in various parts of the body, and cause a variety of emotional—and even spiritual—responses.

GO FOR IT: HOW TO HAVE A G-SPOT ORGASM

All the chapters thus far have technically prepared you to have a G-spot orgasm. You understand the anatomy and how to find the spot. You've got techniques, including plenty of warm-up, deliberate movement, firm pressure, and the "come here" motion. You know about great G-spot toys. You've learned some different intercourse positions to maximize G-spot stimulation. You have the scoop on anal stimulation and how it impacts the G-spot. You've even read some erotic stories to get you in the mood.

RELAX AND LET GO

I recommend just a few more ingredients, and here's an important one: permission. Give yourself permission to have a G-spot orgasm. It may sound strange, but many women hold themselves back from climax. They don't let themselves fully experience pleasure or relax enough to just let go. And a G-spot orgasm really is about letting go.

For one thing, as you increase the G-spot stimulation, the feelings naturally intensify. The pressure may feel overwhelming, like it's just too much—but try to stay with those feelings rather than getting away from them. Take some deep breaths; look into your partner's eyes. Try to ride the wave rather than controlling it. If you want your partner to make an adjustment—faster, deeper, whatever—definitely speak up; you've got to communicate about exactly what you need. But otherwise, give in to the sensations; let them envelop you.

The feeling that you might pee can also ramp up, and an automatic response can kick in. If you have anxiety that you might actually pee, you'll likely tense your pelvic muscles, which is counterproductive to the process. It's the opposite of what you should be doing at this point, and tensing up can throw your orgasm completely off track. Reassure yourself that you're not going to pee. You're not going to pee. Relax into the moment; breathe into it. Let go.

REAL WOMEN, REAL ORGASMS

Here are some real women's descriptions of their G-spot orgasms:

I would describe my G-spot orgasm as a tremendous surge of sensation that wells up within me. The tension in my body builds very fast, and I feel acutely aware of the feeling of the flush on my face as orgasm approaches. It's a deeper-feeling orgasm than others that has a unique and very intense quality. —Emily

A G-spot orgasm feels overwhelming to me. I stop breathing. I can't orgasm again for a while after, unlike with other orgasms. —Elodie

For me, a G-spot orgasm is an ongoing wave of pleasure, complete with plateaus of bliss and peaks of intense self-indulgence. —Missy

A G-spot orgasm feels as if time stands still, and in that timeless moment, I am in sync with my soul, my body, the stars, the moon, the universe. —Ashley

It feels like I'm weightless, unable to breathe, and I have blurred, hazy vision. My arms and legs are useless. I have to wait a while to have another orgasm. And when I work my G-spot and my clit, it's like twice the intensity. —Ina

When I have a G-spot orgasm, I feel a tremendous pressure, a filling up, and then an enormous release. I would almost describe them as uncomfortable, actually. There is definitely a kind of psychological "pushing past" that needs to happen for me to have one, and if any orgasm can bring me to tears, it's this one. And yet, even though they are emotionally satisfying, I can find them physically unsatisfying. The feeling is too diffuse to be truly satisfying. That's the only way I can describe it . . . If I am not too emotionally spent afterward, I typically demand a clitoral orgasm as well, because that physically satisfies me in a way a G-spot orgasm never does. —Nikki

There is no one way to have a G-spot orgasm. For example, you may want to start out with vaginal intercourse in one of the suggested positions, then when you feel close to coming, have your partner switch to using his fingers. That may be what you need to push you over the edge. Or maybe you start with a G-spot toy and work your way up to intercourse. You can build arousal in one of your favorite positions, then change to a position that allows his penis more contact with your G-spot. If you're multiorgasmic, maybe your first orgasm is all about clitoral stimulation to get you aroused, relaxed, and ready for some G-spot play.

IS YOUR FAVORITE POSITION THE BEST ONE FOR G-SPOT ORGASMS?

You've experimented with different positions; you've found some you like and some that have helped you hit the G-spot. What's the best position for a G-spot orgasm? Obviously, this is going to vary from person to person.

Find a position that works well for you and your partner, one that lets your bodies line up best. Pick the position that provides the most pressure on the G-spot. Make sure it's one that gives you and your partner access to all the right parts. Maybe you'd like some extra stimulation on your clitoris or a finger in your anus. Choose a position that is comfortable enough to sustain for a little while—as you build toward coming, you don't want your knees to start hurting or your neck to cramp. Changing positions when you're headed toward an orgasm can break momentum and put you back at square one or close to it. It's all about what feels right for both of you.

Many women develop a routine of coming in a particular position. Some have a surefire position (or two) in which it's easiest for them to have an orgasm. Others can only have an orgasm if they're in one certain position (this often reflects the position you masturbate in). For example, say you come on your back in Missionary most easily. However, traditional Missionary doesn't put enough pressure on your G-spot. Try adapting your go-to position for maximum G-spot stimulation. In this case, put a pillow or Liberator Shape under your butt to change the angle, or fold your legs back toward your shoulders.

Perhaps you've discovered the position that's best for a clitoral orgasm isn't the same as the one that's best for a G-spot orgasm. Find a position that lets you stimulate your clitoris *and* put more direct pressure on your G-spot. (See chapter 7 for suggestions.) Another option is to find a great G-spot position and stay in it until you're about to come, then quickly change to your more reliable orgasm position.

PROLONG THE PLEASURE

Once you've mastered the art of the G-spot orgasm, it's time to take it to the next level. You can intensify your G-spot orgasm by bringing yourself close to orgasm, then decreasing the stimulation and backing off from it. Increase it again until you're close, then back off again. By doing this, you are delaying your orgasm and also teasing it out. The more times you get to the edge but don't go over, the more arousal builds. When you do finally have an orgasm, it's likely to be stronger and longer lasting.

Along the same lines, try to prolong what Masters and Johnson call the plateau phase. This is the time when you're aroused and building toward orgasm. The stimulation can continue, but don't take the next step—increasing pressure on the G-spot or adding clitoral stimulation. Imagine you're keeping your arousal in neutral. It's as if you're at the moment when you want to say, "Harder!" or "Faster!" but instead your partner keeps a steady rhythm. Hold out for as long as you both can in neutral. Then, once you do say, "Harder! Faster!" (or whatever you need to get to that next step), your orgasm will be bigger and better.

REST, RECOVER, REBOUND

Some women have one G-spot orgasm and feel quite satiated. Others are multiorgasmic. The time it takes a woman to recover from an orgasm and become ready for more stimulation varies, but in general women can do it faster than men can. Many women who are easily orgasmic say that once they've had their first G-spot orgasm, they can build back up fairly quickly to another.

Communicate with your partner about what you need. Maybe you want to give yourself a break in between orgasms. Sometimes your G-spot, clitoris, or both are too sensitive for any kind of stimulation right after an orgasm. If the stimulation is temporarily suspended, you can ease back into it when your body feels ready. Some women can keep right on going with penetration or intercourse as long as the direct G-spot stimulation eases up a bit. One orgasm builds on the previous orgasm, like a long, delicious aftershock.

SEXERCISE YOUR BODY

Tone and strengthen your PC muscles by doing Kegel exercises (see the next chapter for specific instructions). As your muscles grow stronger, you can deliberately contract them during penetration by tightening around whatever is inside you—a finger, toy, or penis. Using these muscles increases blood flow to the area, brings your awareness and focus to your entire genital region, and pumps up the volume of your orgasm.

CHAPTER 11

YOU MAKE ME GUSH: FEMALE EJACULATION

It's not something that I notice during sex, but I know I have a tendency to squirt after sex. I don't really feel it much, except for the fluid that starts dripping down my thighs.

—Ava

Increasing waves come that cause me to tighten my PC muscles, until I finally let go and feel a release that causes squirting.

—Lee

Female ejaculation is fun, it feels good, and it's another way women can experience pleasure. For some, the sensations that come with female ejaculation are entirely unique. Some women say it feels like an intense release. Others ejaculate and orgasm at the same time, creating a wet, wonderful climax that both partners can enjoy.

Some women already ejaculate, without trying to do it or without necessarily knowing anything about it. Often, they or their partners are confused about what is happening—they may believe something is wrong or think they're peeing. Many women have reported feeling confused, embarrassed, or shameful about their ejaculations, especially those who had no knowledge about female ejaculation prior to doing it. Some have been so mortified that they have avoided sex or stopped themselves from having orgasms in order to prevent ejaculating again. Some discussed it with doctors who've told them they're incontinent.

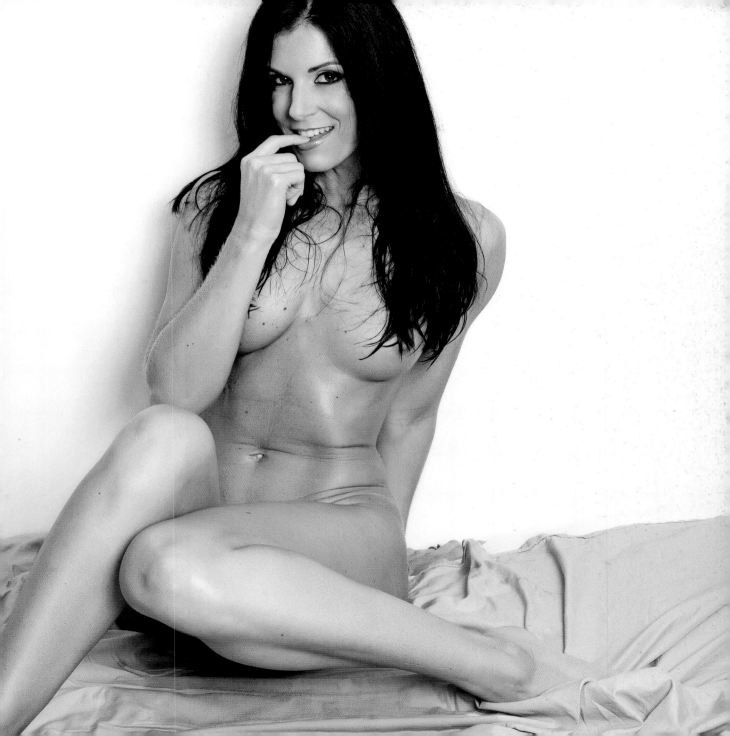

Putting the correct information about female ejaculation out into the world can reassure women who already do it that it's normal and healthy and they are not alone. In one study, Amy L. Gilliland concluded that, "Familiarity with ejaculation before experiencing it personally led to greater acceptance of the phenomena."[12] Validating women's diverse sexual expression and experience is critical to our self-knowledge, self-confidence, and empowerment.

Do you recall a sexual experience during which you may have ejaculated, but just aren't sure? Or maybe you want to find out how to recreate that experience again. If you've never experienced female ejaculation, you may have heard about it from a friend, seen it in an adult film, or been curious to discover what it's all about. With education, you can learn how it works and how to do it, expanding your erogenous zones and adding to your erotic repertoire in the process. Remember, this discussion of female ejaculation is focused on validating experience and learning about our bodies and pleasure. It's not meant to make *anyone* feel as if she's missing out or having inferior sex and orgasms just because she doesn't ejaculate.

WHAT IS FEMALE EJACULATION?

A lot of confusion and misinformation still exist about female ejaculation. Some people believe it's not even possible. But I've seen hundreds of women ejaculate, and I know it's real.

Female ejaculation is not a new phenomenon, although from the mainstream media you'd think it was something we've just "discovered." Widespread public awareness of female ejaculation and its role in female pleasure is fairly recent. Grafenberg, for whom the G-spot was named, was the first to mention female ejaculation in a scientific journal in the 1950s.

INTRODUCING FEMALE EJACULATION

Research about this "phenomenon" began to appear in the late 1970s, and was expanded on in the early 1980s in the groundbreaking book *The G-Spot*. However, researchers have found centuries-old references to female ejaculation in medical literature, sex studies, and historical texts.

Since the publication of *The G-Spot*, fewer than forty studies about female ejaculation have been published. Because of varied methodology, small samples of women in the studies, and even researcher bias, we have no definitive or conclusive information about female ejaculation. Plenty of anecdotal evidence exists, however, along with several strong qualitative studies and some promising physiological research that when some women masturbate and/or have sex with a partner, they ejaculate fluid before, during, or after orgasm. The bottom line is: We still don't know enough about this area of female sexuality.

WHERE DOES THE FLUID COME FROM?

As discussed in previous chapters, there are glands embedded within the urethral sponge. Among the approximately thirty paraurethral glands, the Skene's glands are the two that adjoin the anterior wall of the vagina.[13] Some researchers believe the Skene's glands produce female ejaculate.

Whether it is solely the province of the Skene's glands or other glands also get into the act, the glands fill with fluid when a woman becomes aroused, and the urethral sponge begins to swell. The swelling is what makes the G-spot more prominent and more sensitive to stimulation. Most researchers believe that the fluid is expelled from the glands into the paraurethral ducts, moves from the ducts into the urethra, and then comes out the urethra. This is supported by what actual women report—they describe a buildup of pressure in the area of the G-spot followed by fluid expulsion. The fluid is different from vaginal lubrication and from urine. The expulsion is called female ejaculation, also known as vaginal ejaculation or squirting.

WHAT, EXACTLY, IS SHE SQUIRTING?

That brings us to one of the most common assumptions that people make: Women are peeing, not ejaculating. After all, the fluid comes out of the urethra, just as urine does. But there is compelling evidence that the fluid is *not* urine. Several studies have shown that female ejaculatory fluid contains prostatic specific antigen (PSA) markers that are similar to PSA markers in prostatic fluid and semen produced by the prostate in men; these same markers are not found in urine.[14] Because the G-spot has been likened to the male prostate in many different ways, it makes sense that both structures would produce a similar fluid.

Five different studies show the majority of women's ejaculate contains zero or low levels of urea and creatinine, both of which are found in urine. Ejaculate also tests positive for prostatic acid phosphatase (PAP), which is found in male prostatic fluid and has higher amounts of glucose than urine does. Other studies have registered no significant difference between urine and ejaculate, or have had inconclusive results. Some attribute the presence of urea in female ejaculate to trace amounts of urea from urine residue in the urethra. Others conclude that female ejaculate may contain some urine but is not only urine.[15]

You can do your own research, if you like. If you or your female partner has ever ejaculated, look at the ejaculate, smell it, taste it. You'll likely see that the fluid appears watery and clear. It may taste odorless or salty or sweet depending on where a woman is in her menstrual cycle.

FROM DRIBBLE TO GUSH: COMPLEXITIES AND VARIABLES

The reason ejaculation is so hard to measure is that different women ejaculate in very different ways. Lots of variables contribute to the confusion. Most prominently, some women ejaculate every time they have sex, some do it once in a while, and some never ejaculate—and there is no definitive answer about why. Some women ejaculate exclusively from G-spot stimulation, others from only clitoral stimulation, others a combination . . . you get the picture.

Some women shoot the ejaculate out of their bodies in a dramatic, amazing way. For others, the fluid sort of dribbles or leaks out, leaving them with a puddle under their butts. It may not be as visually showy, but they are still ejaculating. Still others fall somewhere in between, delivering ejaculatory fluid in spurts or gushes, depending on the situation.

Some women ejaculate a small amount, whereas others can ejaculate a lot of fluid. Based on research reported in *The G-Spot*, Ladas, Whipple, and Perry estimated that women could ejaculate from a few drops up to ¼ teaspoon (1.3 ml).[16]

HISTORIC AND SLANG TERMS

Female Ejaculation

Squirting

Gushing

Vaginal ejaculation

Vajaculation

Geyser of love (Dr. Susan Block)[21]

Wet orgasm

Ejaculatory Fluid

Amrita (India)[22]

Liquor vitae (ancient Rome)[23]

Girl jizz

Girl juice

Nectar of Aphrodite (ancient Greece)

Semen of women (Kama Sutra)[24]

The third water (China)[25]

In later research, Beverly Whipple insisted it's not possible to expel more than ⅔ to 1 teaspoon (3 to 5 ml). Subsequent studies have reported amounts ranging from ½ teaspoon to 10 teaspoons, or ⅕ cup (3 to 50 ml).[17]

Female ejaculation expert and author Deborah Sundahl says that in a single ejaculation, women can release anywhere from 2 tablespoons (30 ml) to 1 cup (235 ml) of fluid.

From less than 1 teaspoon (5 ml) all the way up to 1 cup (235 ml) is quite a range. Researchers can't agree on how much fluid the glands are capable of producing and how it is that women can expel large amounts. Many researchers agree with one of Gilliland's conclusions: "While small amounts of fluid may be produced by the female prostate, logic says that large amounts of fluid must be stored and released from the bladder."[18] Plus, some women are multiple ejaculators; they squirt once, then can be stimulated to squirt again, and in some cases, several more times.

WHY DO ONLY SOME WOMEN EJACULATE?

We don't have a clear explanation for why some women are frequent ejaculators, some never do it, and others do it occasionally or only when a particular kind of stimulation occurs. According to a paper published in *Nurse Practioner* of women's reports of female ejaculation, from 14 to 54 percent of women have reported at least one experience of ejaculating.[19] So what about the rest?

One theory suggests that every woman does ejaculate, but many women ejaculate such a small amount of fluid that it's not very noticeable or can be chalked up to vaginal juices, personal lubricants, or even sweat. Another theory says that all women's bodies create the fluid, but for some, it is never expelled; instead, they experience retrograde ejaculation, during which the fluid travels back to the bladder. It may be possible that when some women pee immediately after sex, they ejaculate the fluid into the toilet (or ejaculate and pee at the same time).

Two research studies by Giulia D'Amati, Emmanuelle Jannini, and their colleagues—one in 2003 at Sapienza University of Rome and another at L'Aquila University in central Italy published in 2006—attribute the variables to actual anatomical differences in women. They propose that the existence and size of the ducts that connect the Skene's glands to the urethra can vary greatly among women. If the ducts are the conduit for ejaculate excreted from the glands, then differences in the size and number of ducts—or their absence altogether—may explain why some women ejaculate and others don't.[20]

Because the ability, method, frequency, quantity, and repetition of ejaculation can vary dramatically from woman to woman (and some women don't do it at all), it's wide open for criticism and controversy. I choose to believe the studies I've read about female ejaculation that support the experiences of the thousands of women I've met over the years who ejaculate.

THE KAMA SUTRA AND FEMALE EJACULATION

In her book *Female Ejaculation and the G-Spot: Not Your Mother's Orgasm Book*, Deborah Sundahl notes that the Kama Sutra, written more than two millennia ago, discusses female ejaculation. Its author, the yogic sage Vatsyayana, writes, "The semen of women continues to fall from the beginning of the sexual union to its end, and in the same way as that of the male."

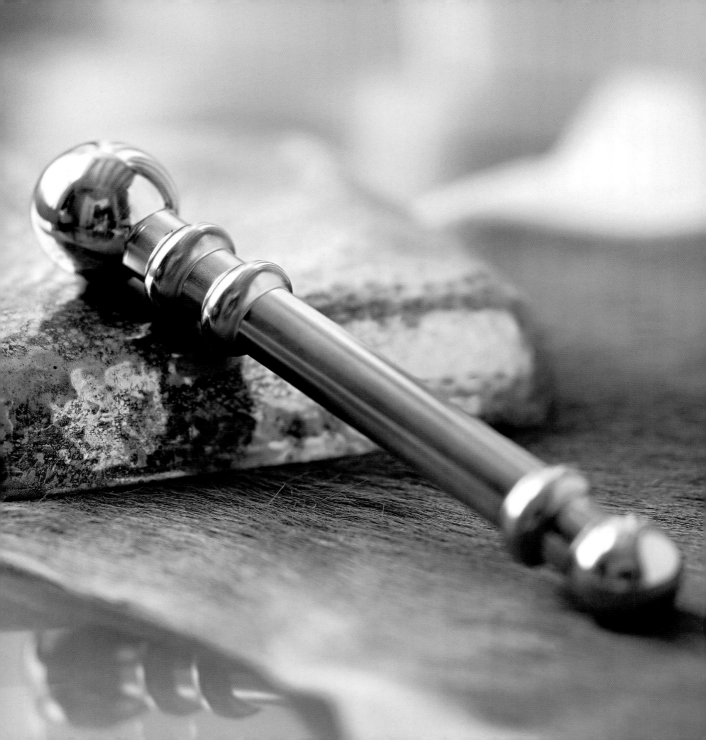

TRISTAN'S TOP PICKS FOR KEGEL EXERCISING

These also make great sex toys for penetration and G-spot stimulation!

BETTY'S BARBELL: This stainless steel barbell designed by masturbation guru Dr. Betty Dodson weighs about 1 pound (450 g). The weight and solid feel of this barbell offer the most resistance of any of these toys.

JUNO WEIGHTED PELVIC EXERCISER: This is a smooth, seamless, Lucite wand from The Berman Center sex toy line. Metal balls embedded in the Lucite graduate in girth and weight.

ENERGIE: This hard plastic Kegel exerciser from Natural Contours has a gentle curve on each end (different from the first two, which are straight), and the ends are slightly bulbous.

PREPARING TO GUSH

Ladas, Whipple, and Perry were among the first to argue in *The G-Spot* that there is a link between the strength of your PC muscles and female ejaculation. Actually, your PC muscles play a big role in the overall health of your vagina and the pleasure you experience during sexual activity of any kind. As I mentioned earlier, your PC muscles are a group of broad, flat muscles at the bottom of the pelvic floor. They are an important part of sexual anatomy because they support the pelvis from the pubic bone to the tailbone; they support the clitoral structure, vagina, and anus. Healthy PC muscles can increase the vagina's lubricating ability and make your entire genital region more responsive to stimulation.

If you've ever seen or heard about a woman who can "shoot" her ejaculate—really propel it from her body—it's likely that she has strong, well-developed PC muscles that give her good control over her ejaculation. Weaker PC muscles may account for the dribbling that other women experience when they ejaculate. Women with very tense or atrophied PC muscles may not be able to ejaculate at all. It's quite common for the PC muscles to be weakened after pregnancy and birth, surgery, a long period of celibacy, or as part of the natural aging process. So, your first step toward learning to squirt and having a squirting orgasm is to tone your PC muscles.

KEGEL EXERCISES FOR YOUR PC MUSCLES

Kegel exercises—named for Arnold Kegel, the gynecologist who invented pelvic floor muscle exercises as well as a tool to measure muscle strength—tone your PC muscles. To find your PC muscles, pretend you're peeing and want to stop the flow of urine. The muscles you tighten are your PC muscles. You can also experiment with using a dildo during masturbation. Try to squeeze the dildo with your vagina. The more difficult it is to do, the weaker your muscles. Here are some basic exercises:

IN AND EX: Relax your body and bring your awareness to your genitals. Take several deep breaths. Take another deep breath and this time, while you inhale, contract the muscles and hold the contraction for a few seconds. Then exhale and relax the muscles. Start by trying to do this twenty times. For best results, slowly work your way up to about a hundred repetitions per day in one sitting.

IN AND TEN: Relax your body and bring your awareness to your genitals. Take several deep breaths. On your next breath, inhale deeply, and as you do, tighten and release the muscles repeatedly (about ten times). Then exhale and relax. Try to do these contractions quickly. Over time, gradually increase the amount of sets you do (one set being one inhalation with ten contractions). I recommend doing twenty to fifty sets a day.

IN-HOLD AND EX-PUSH: Relax your body and bring your awareness to your genitals. Take several deep breaths. When you inhale next, contract your muscles as if you were trying to suck something inside your vagina and anus. Then exhale and gently bear down, pushing out that object. This combination will exercise your pelvic muscles and your stomach muscles. For best results, do ten to thirty each day.

KEGELS WITH TOYS

After you have mastered these exercises, take your strengthening routine to the next level by adding resistance. Ben Wa balls (popular brand names include Luna Beads and Smartballs) are two balls about the size of golf balls; another style uses just one ball. Larger balls are better for beginners—you can graduate to a smaller size once you've developed your PC muscles. The balls are usually made of hard plastic or plastic coated with silicone. They may be separate or connected with a loop at one end for easier insertion and retrieval. You can purchase them at better sex toy stores and websites.

1. Spread some lube on the balls, and then slide them inside your vagina.

2. Try the "In and Ex" exercise.

3. As you inhale, feel your muscles grip the balls; when you exhale, release your hold on the balls.

You'll also find dildos, wands, and barbells designed specifically for Kegel exercises. They are made of a hard material and, like the balls, provide resistance during the exercises. Be sure to warm yourself up for penetration before you begin.

1. When you're ready, slide the well-lubed toy inside your vagina. Many of them have two different-size ends; you want to start with the larger end, which is easier to work with than the smaller end.

2. Begin with the "In and Ex" exercise.

3. See how much of a grip you can get on the toy—can you actually move it with your muscles?

The more you do the exercises, the more you'll be able to squeeze the toy. This can also come in handy later when you practice squeezing your partner's penis during intercourse, a sensation that drives some men wild.

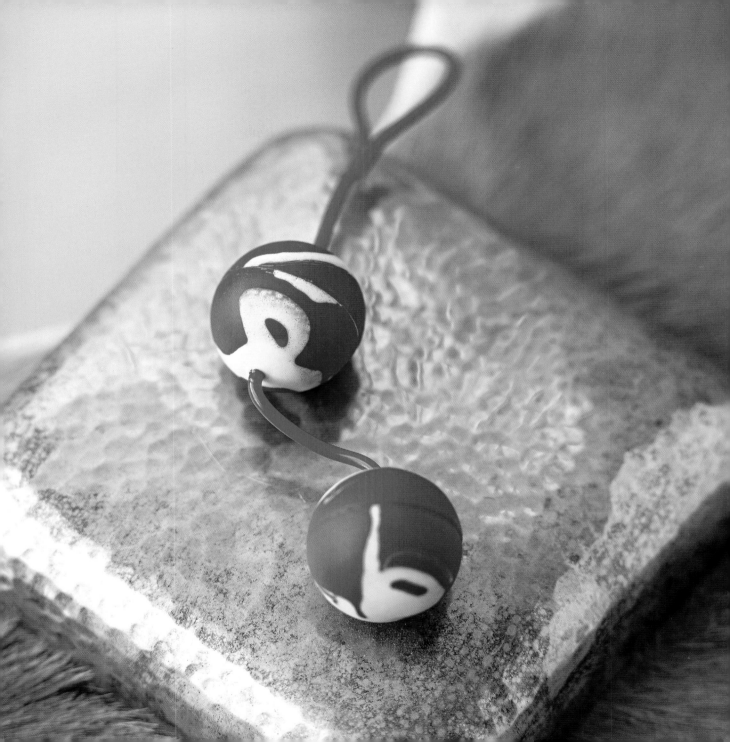

CHAPTER 12

LEARN TO EJACULATE: EXPERIENCE FULL-BODY SATISFACTION

I usually ejaculate several times, sometimes without really feeling that I've come, as part of a buildup to a string of larger orgasms. It feels like a spray of water leaving my pussy! It doesn't feel like urinating. It's pleasurable, especially when there's a cock (or similar) butting up against my G-spot, and I can feel the outward flow of energy. My pussy then feels more relaxed and "marshy" wet, and the relaxation spreads into my hips and pelvis, too. The bed sheets do get ridiculously wet.

—Penny

As I discussed in the chapter on G-spot orgasms, the first step to ejaculating is to give yourself permission. Female ejaculation includes a very strong emotional and psychological component. You need to relax and go with the flow. This also means letting go of fear and anxiety. If you're tense or anxious, chances are you won't ejaculate. Some women struggle with receiving pleasure and letting go in the moment. Past experiences, insecurities, and bottled-up feelings can hold you back from experiencing your full sexual potential. Tell yourself that your body is wonderful the way it is. Ignore the voices in your head that may say ejaculation is weird or abnormal. Don't hide this unique part of you. Embrace your sexual power and celebrate it.

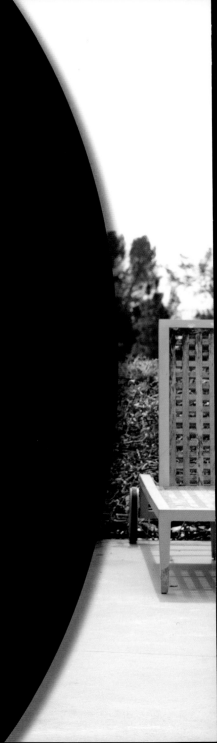

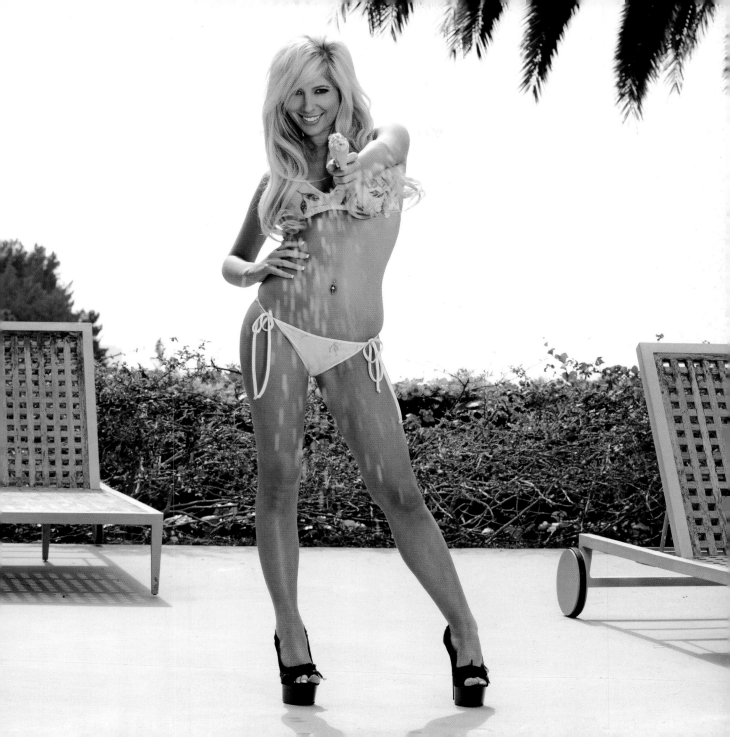

LEARNING TO SQUIRT

If you'd like to ejaculate, first make sure you are hydrated. As you can imagine, dehydration affects the production of all kinds of fluids in our bodies. Many women I know who ejaculate say that if they haven't had enough to drink or are dehydrated from exercise or something else, they have a more difficult time ejaculating or they ejaculate much less fluid.

Before you try to ejaculate, you should definitely be sure to pee. It's a good idea to empty your bladder before sex anyway, but in this case, a trip to the bathroom will reassure you that you're not going to pee, which is a common fear that holds women back. Keep in mind that in this sense women are very similar to men: When very aroused, they often can't pee at all—but they can ejaculate.

1. As you (if you're self-stimulating) or your partner intensifies G-spot stimulation, you will feel like you really need to pee. This is the point when some women just stop altogether and say the pressure and sensations are "too much" or overwhelming. Or you may automatically clench your PC muscles—the muscles that stop the flow of urine—and it may not even be a conscious response on your part.

2. When the urge to pee gets really strong, when the stimulation feels overwhelming and you want to stop is precisely when you need to *keep going*. Remind yourself that you peed before sex and you aren't going to pee now.

3. Take some deep breaths and let yourself go with the sensations.

4. If you feel yourself start to clamp those muscles, take charge and do the opposite: Relax and bear down like you're trying to push something out of your vagina. Remember your Kegel exercises, especially the "In-Pull, Ex-Push," and practice that. Keep relaxing and pushing out. If the stars are aligned properly, you should ejaculate.

What does ejaculation feel like? Some women are very aware of exactly when they are ejaculating, and the moment it first begins. They feel like they have to pee, a sensation of pressure builds, they relax and bear down, and they release ejaculatory fluid. Other women are surprised to find out they ejaculated when they discover a puddle under their butts. The more often you ejaculate, the more conscious you will become of what is happening, and when it happens. The more you relax and stay connected to your body, the better you'll be able to gauge how the ejaculation process works for you.

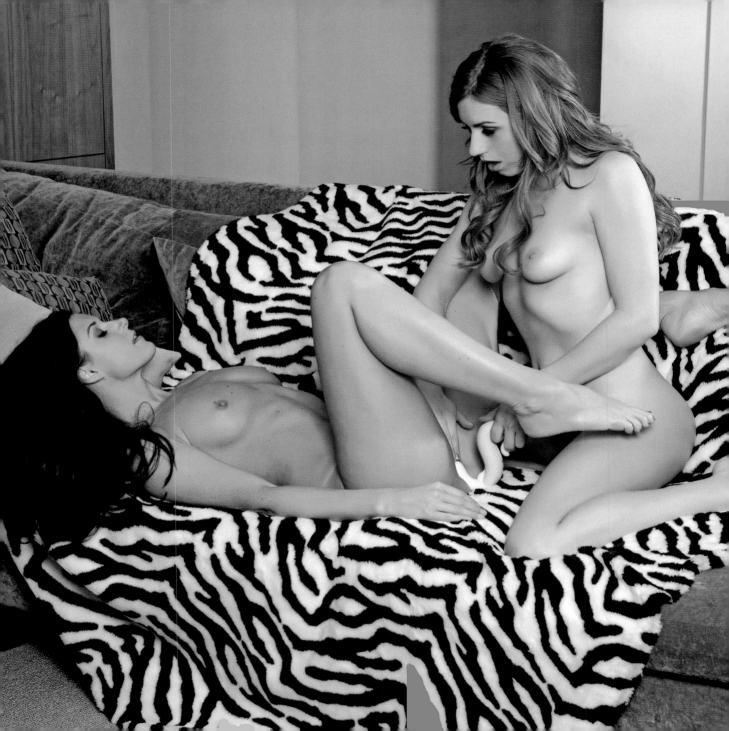

HOW TO HELP YOUR PARTNER EJACULATE

For many women, intense, prolonged G-spot stimulation is what gets them to ejaculate. So your first stop on the road to female ejaculation is the G-spot.

1. Use your fingers to find the spot against the front wall of the vagina.

2. Move your fingers toward the front of her body and down slightly as if you're saying "come here." It's almost like you are trying to pull the G-spot out of her.

3. Feel it begin to swell underneath your fingers as you stimulate it.

4. Keep going, with consistent, powerful pressure. Or use one of the many toys designed especially for the G-spot. The key, as with other kinds of stimulation, is to build the intensity—don't go too hard too quickly.

5. Some women prefer G-spot stimulation by itself, whereas others want clitoral stimulation as well. Because all the nerves and tissues are connected, they play off one other, helping stimulate the entire area. Add some clit stimulation if she wants it.

6. As you continue G-spot stimulation, you'll feel the textured area on the front wall swell even more.

7. In some women, you can also hear a very distinct "sloshing" sound. It's markedly different from the sound of penetration; it's juicier and louder.

8. Keep up the stimulation. Experienced ejaculators often know right before it happens and may tell you when they're ready to squirt. Others may not know, but you may feel them start to bear down and push out.

9. Now you have a couple of options. Keep doing what you're doing, then give the sponge one good pull. Or use your fingers to actually press firmly up on the front wall.

⟲ TRISTAN'S TIPS

This is very important: If you're using more than two fingers, a dildo, or penis, it's likely you could be blocking the urethral opening. That means you're blocking the ejaculate's escape route. If this is the case, when she tells you or you think she's ready to squirt, move whatever's in the way out of her vagina—some women can actually use their muscles to push you out. Once the urethral opening is no longer blocked, the ejaculate is free to come out.

EJACULATION DURING INTERCOURSE

So, what about intercourse—with a penis or a strap-on dildo—and female ejaculation? Remember that vaginal intercourse is not always the ideal method for G-spot stimulation; consequently, it's often not the best way to make a woman ejaculate. Experiment with the positions discussed in chapter 7.

- Positions such as Yab-Yum, Horizontal Tailgate, and Inverted Spider may prove too awkward to make squirting easy, unless your partner can squirt while you're still inside her.

- In Missionary Fold position (where she lies on her back with her legs up, either folded back and against her shoulders or on her partner's shoulders), you can communicate easily and she can tell you when she's ready so you can pull out.

- In Doggie Style (with her head and shoulders down and you behind her), you can access her G-spot and work it well with deliberate strokes.

- In Stallion (Doggie Style, but with just you standing), use your extra thrusting power to put more pressure on her G-spot.

- In Cowgirl position (where she's on top facing you), she can ride your penis until the moment she feels ready to explode, then she can raise herself slightly, and let the ejaculate spray all over you.

- The same holds true for Reverse Chairman (with you sitting in a chair and her on your lap facing away with her feet on the floor), which may be a better angle depending on the curve of the penis or dildo.

EJACULATION WITHOUT DIRECT G-SPOT STIMULATION

Many researchers have investigated and proposed a direct link between G-spot stimulation and female ejaculation.

For many women, direct G-spot stimulation is the key to ejaculating. But not for *all* women. Some women can ejaculate from clitoral stimulation alone, without any penetration or G-spot stimulation at all. In fact, for some, clitoral stimulation is the only way they can ejaculate. In Amy Gilliland's 2001–2002 study of thirteen women, published in the journal *Sexuality & Culture* in 2009, the majority of the women she interviewed said they had ejaculated through clitoral stimulation alone.

How can we explain this in light of all the information we have connecting the G-spot to female ejaculation? The G-spot may not be the only trigger point that causes the glands in the urethral sponge to fill with fluid. Some experts say when you stimulate the vulva (which includes the clitoral hood and glans), you can stimulate the external part of the urethral sponge—specifically the area around the urethral opening, which in turn stimulates the glands in the sponge to produce fluid. Others contend that the G-spot is part of the complex clitoral structure; therefore, stimulating the external parts of the clitoris will also stimulate the internal parts, including the G-spot. That stimulation can be enough to cause the glands to fill with fluid and release the fluid.

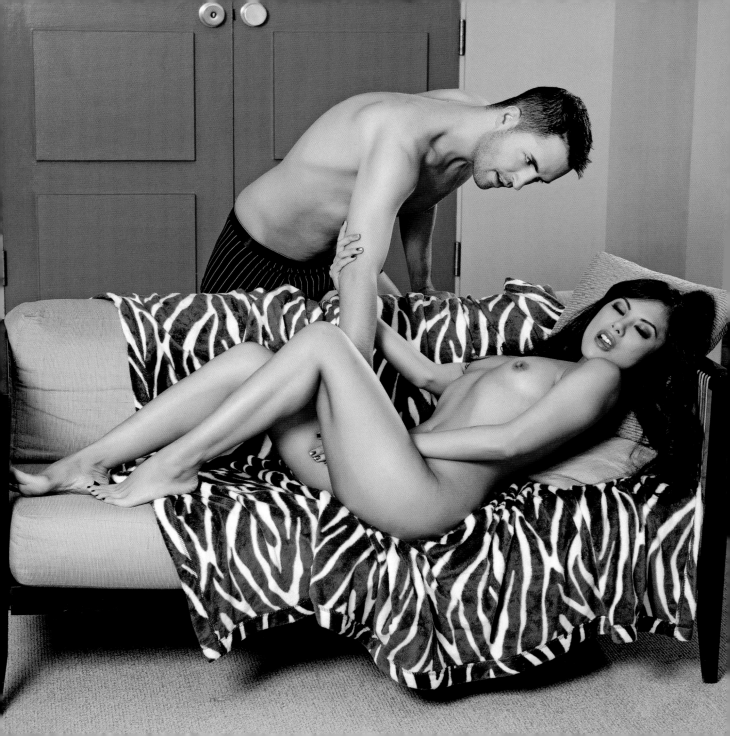

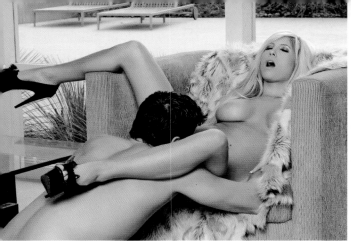
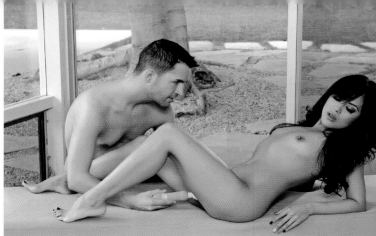

EJACULATION EXERCISE

1. If you'd like to try to ejaculate without internal G-spot stimulation, begin by stimulating your clitoris as you usually do.

2. Then, with your hand, your partner's tongue or fingers, or a vibrator, try to spread out the stimulation. Instead of concentrating on and around the clitoral glans and hood, add stimulation to the entire vulva, including the area around the urethral opening. This is where a vibrator with a large head or one with plenty of surface area works to your advantage—you can stimulate a lot more of the vulva with it.

3. If you start to feel the urge to pee, you're headed in the right direction.

4. Keep up the stimulation and pay attention to how the sensations may differ from when you target just the clitoris.

5. Or you can try intensifying your clitoral stimulation. Some women say that when they are very aroused and add vigorous clitoral stimulation, they are more likely to ejaculate.

WHAT WOMEN ARE SAYING: CLITORAL STIMULATION AND FEMALE EJACULATION

Here's what two women say about clitoral stimulation and female ejaculation:

I don't ejaculate when I masturbate, but I do when a lover is going down on me. I guess it's the enhanced arousal of being with someone. Luckily, my lovers have always really enjoyed it—I have one who describes the way I "flood" him as one of his favorite things about having sex with me. —Pam

For me, squirting is not necessarily orgasmic—it often accompanies orgasm but sometimes comes before or after, or completely independently. What gets me there is very intense clitoral stimulation; G-spot stuff doesn't do it. In fact, having anything in my vagina at all usually prevents me from ejaculating. The feeling is one of intense, deep tickling inside that eventually releases in pulses. —Jane

ANAL PENETRATION AND EJACULATION

Some women can also ejaculate as a result of anal penetration. As discussed in chapter 8, the G-spot can be indirectly stimulated, especially in certain positions, during anal sex. If you enjoy anal penetration and feel you get pretty intense G-spot sensations from it, you may be able to ejaculate. Find that position where you feel the most pressure on the front wall of your vagina. If you want more stimulation, perhaps slip a finger or toy inside your vagina to increase the pressure. When you start to experience the urge to pee, don't stop, keep going. Relax your pelvic muscles and bear down. You just might find that it will make you gush!

COME AND SQUIRT: EXPERIENCE A FULL-BODY ORGASM

For some women, female ejaculation does not necessarily happen at the same time as an orgasm; it may happen before or after instead. For them, ejaculation can feel like a big release, but it's not a type of orgasm. Others ejaculate simultaneously with orgasm and say that a squirting orgasm feels entirely unique. Some describe it as a deeper, full-body orgasm or an intense release of muscle tension after which they feel completely satisfied and exhausted.

Not only can a squirting orgasm feel fantastic for some, but it can also answer the age-old question, "Did you come?" Men (and some women) can be perplexed about the female orgasm because they are not sure whether their partners are actually having one. Sure, there are noises, moans, and muscle contractions, but, they say, there is no definitive way to know when a woman has climaxed. When a woman has an orgasm with ejaculation, there is a clear visual sign, which can be a big turn-on for both the women who do it and their partners. You can't fake female ejaculation! Plus, some folks love all that wetness. It's erotic for them to be entirely uninhibited about sharing body fluids. If you like to feel fluids on your hands, on your legs, even on your face, then female ejaculation can provide plenty of warm, wet goodness.

KEYS TO HAVING SQUIRTING ORGASMS

If you'd like to have squirting orgasms, make sure you've been doing your Kegel exercises. Strong PC muscles will help you have better control over both orgasm and female ejaculation. If direct G-spot stimulation has made you ejaculate in the past, then continue on that path. Practice the techniques discussed earlier:

1. Do lots of warm-up followed by vigorous G-spot stimulation.

2. Relax.

3. Push past the urge to pee.

4. Let go, and push out.

5. To intensify the sensations, try adding clitoral stimulation to the mix.

6. If you let go and nothing comes out, go back to the G-spot stimulation and work your way back up.

7. Listen for that distinct sloshing sound; when you hear it, try again to bear down, using your muscles to push.

If you've squirted via clitoral stimulation or anal penetration, then focus on that. Feel the pressure building inside you. When you feel like you're on the edge of an orgasm, repeat your method for squirting: Relax your body, remind yourself you're not going to pee, breathe through the intense feelings, bear down, and the fluid should come.

Remember that you may not come and ejaculate simultaneously the first time you try. As with most things, practice, practice, practice. You may not be able to do it at all; for you, squirting and coming may be two different experiences. That's okay. Don't be hard on yourself about any of it. Accept and embrace what works for you and how your body responds.

THE WET SPOT: CLEANUP TIPS FOR SQUIRTERS

If you have experienced the pleasure and amazement of female ejaculation, you probably already know that it can be, well, wet. And wet is wonderful, except that washing your sheets every time you have sex is not. Here are a few tips for you old pros as well as those of you who are considering getting into it. Having a plan for handling the squirt means less laundry, and no one has to sleep in the wet spot (and trust me, that spot can be bigger than you imagine).

If you are not expecting a tidal wave, slide a towel underneath you to catch the fluid. However, if you are a medium to heavy sheet soaker, I recommend some better supplies. Disposable absorbent bed pads for incontinent people are sold in most drugstores and medical supply stores; in hospitals, these handy pads are called "chucks." Chucks are sheets with absorbent material on one side and plastic on the other. They're great for soaking up all that girl jizz, and you just throw them away when you are done.

WHAT WOMEN ARE SAYING: EJACULATING ORGASMS

Here's how three different women describe their ejaculating orgasms:

When I am having my G-spot stimulated it begins by feeling like . . . oooh, then slowly starts to feel more raw, more animalistic. I cannot control my hips from trying to get whatever is inside me to rub me more vigorously. At climax, I get that "I'm going to pee!" sensation. The only way I can continue with the orgasm is to clear my head at that moment and just let go. When I am unable to let go, I still have an orgasm but will not ejaculate and am left feeling just okay. If I ejaculate, I am left feeling complete and fulfilled. —Tina

G-spot orgasms seem to be more muscular, in comparison to clitoral orgasms that seem to be all about concentrated nerve endings—no less satisfying, but definitely in a different way. It feels like every ounce of blood goes to that area, and every muscle is flexed and waiting for the release. I'm a gusher, so the release is quite tangible to me and my partner. The best part is that they can keep going and going . . . with round after round. Since all my muscles are flexed and my energy is focused, I often forget to breathe when I'm actually coming . . . I get lightheaded and a true "afterglow" ensues. —Jules

I need to have clitoral stimulation and penetration for my squirting orgasms. A squirting O has become the only orgasm I want to have! For me, my squirting orgasms are an intense surge that starts at my amazing clitoris, goes up my spine, and clogs my head! It is the most incredible feeling I've ever felt in my life. —Erin

If you are more environmentally conscious, you may want to try a reusable, washable, diaper-changing pad. These are sold anywhere you find baby and crib supplies. (I suggest looking for one that has the least amount of baby stuff printed on it.) Usually, they consist of a plastic pad with an absorbent cover that you can remove and toss in the washing machine. Serious squirters may need something a little more durable with more coverage to protect not just the sheet but also the mattress underneath it. In this case, look for a waterproof (not water-resistant) mattress cover. In the old days, they were made entirely of plastic, which made lots of noise when you rolled around and didn't exactly inspire sexy nights. Now, you'll find fabric mattress covers that protect your mattress without producing a crinkly sound underneath you.

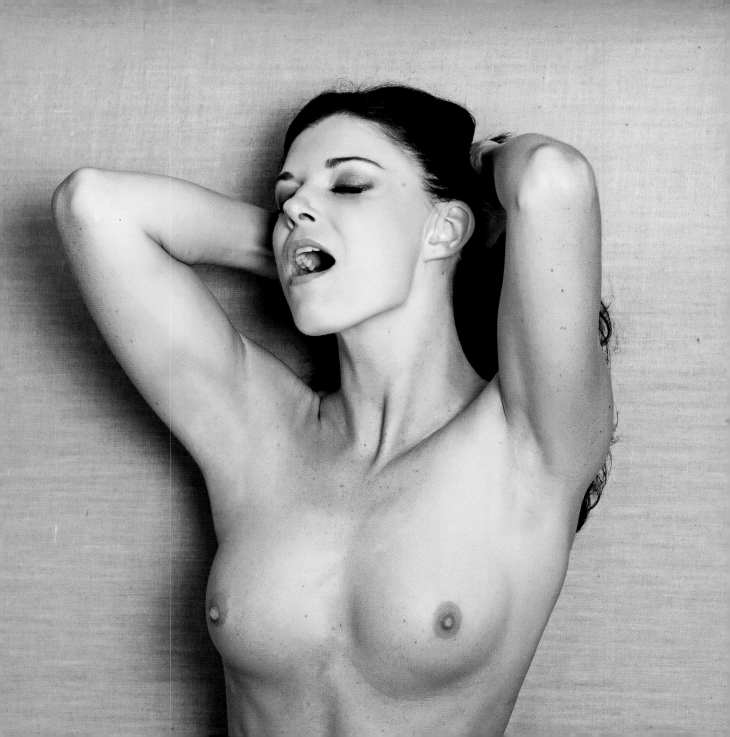

CHAPTER 13

EROTIC INTERLUDE #3: "FLY"

BY VALERIE ALEXANDER

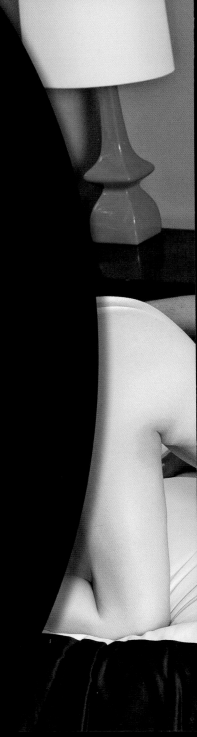

It's night on Neverland. The lost boys sit around the fire. Their war-painted faces glow with the fervor of boyhood delusion. They want adventure; their throats ache with unsung cries of battle and bloodlust. But the night won't begin until Peter arrives. Restless and agitated, the boys open beers and throw sticks into the fire and wait for him to return from his latest girl, his latest flight.

Across the island, Tigerlily also dreams of Peter. Naked on her bed, she toys with her tight amber tits, one fingertip circling her nipples. The other hand surfs down the silky dip of her navel until she cradles her own pussy under the pretense of someone else's touch. She is beautiful but she is ignored. Her clit hardens to the dream of something ambiguous, fantasies of a pointy-faced boy who at eighteen is all swagger and brashness. A boy whose thick golden-red hair is always askew, whose clever eyes are always alive with the possibility of danger. He is lithe and he is pretty, and from spying on him in the lake, she knows he is well endowed. But it's not his cock that haunts her dreams; it's his smile. He's a beautiful boy with a beautiful smile. All the girls want Peter.

Tigerlily wants to fuck him more than life itself, but she wants more than that; she wants to pin him down and rub her pussy all over his face until he surrenders completely, until his endless taunts and stories are silenced. She wants to break his will and slap his face, wants to subsume his bragging in her sexual heat. Yet mostly what she wants is for Peter to teach her to fly. But he won't. Girls don't fly in Peter's world, not unless it's by holding on to him.

She rolls her clit between her fingers, slowly rubbing as she imagines that she is him. Now she's climbing rocks and scaling pirate ships, a prettier daredevil than he as she levitates with her long black hair flowing behind her like a flag. She knifes through the dark violet sky over Neverland until she sees Peter's last lover walking out of the lake. The girl is naked in the starlight and voluptuous, as Peter likes his women to be. She's smiling dreamily as she towels off, perhaps lost in a reverie of that narrow-hipped boy who fucked her so soundly and never returned.

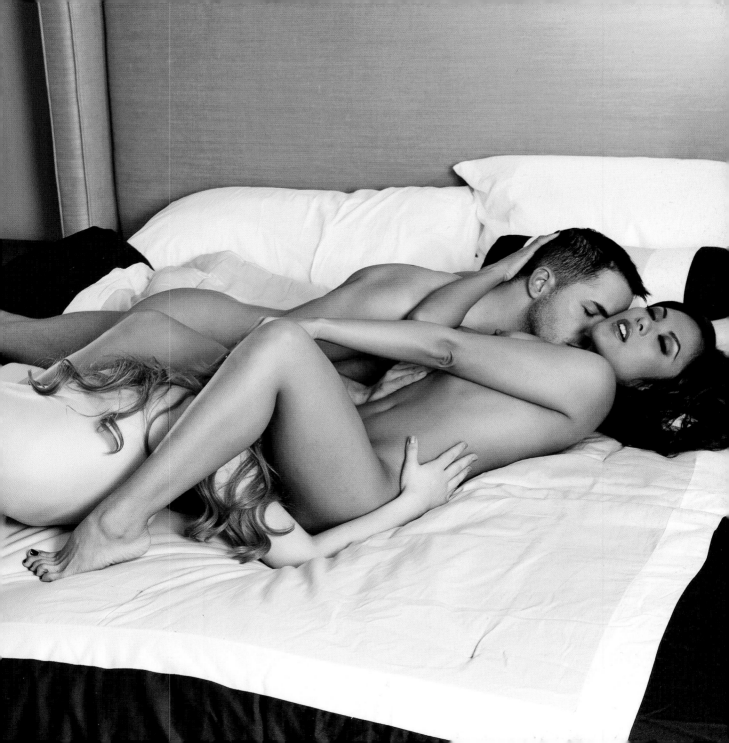

"I'll fuck you better than he ever will," Tigerlily mutters and swoops down, still in her Peter guise, to push the girl down against the sand. Roughly she spreads her legs and fucks her with Peter's cock, pumping into her with savage thrusts.

"I knew you'd come back, Peter," the girl groans, arching her spine. "Oh, harder . . . "

But he never will come back, Tigerlily thinks as her interest in the scene abruptly dies. She changes the fantasy to the last actual time she saw Peter, digging ammunition out of a pirate ship. Cheekbones smeared with dirt, bare-chested in ripped jeans, he talked excitedly of a fight he had won the previous night. She had been wearing her shortest dress, flexing her long bare legs for him. But he was too wrapped up in his story to even look at her.

But if he had. If he had turned and really seen her, the most hot-blooded girl on the island, he just might have knelt between her legs. Pushing her dress up her thighs, he would have pushed his thumb deep into her pussy, making her squirm there on the ship deck . . .

The thought sends a white bolt of heat ricocheting through her body, her cunt shuddering over and over around her fingers. Wetness soaks her hand, her thighs, as she furiously rubs herself into another flood of contractions. "I'm going to fuck you," Tigerlily whispers, her legs spread wide for that phantom Peter thrusting into her. "I'm going to fuck you blind."

Collapsing back on her pillow, she licks the tangy, pearly strands of honey from each finger. Then she gets up and throws on her dress and heads off into the night.

The lost boys are still waiting to be found tonight by the boy they call their leader. Past the empty beer bottles and the boastful tales of girls fucked and discarded, their thoughts are anxious. They are not warriors or lovers, just followers still.

And then suddenly there he is at the fire with a self-satisfied smile. By the hand he holds his latest conquest: a hesitant-looking girl of about eighteen, softer than his usual girls and doe-eyed, her long brown hair wet and disheveled. She has the dazed and startled look of someone who has flown for the first time.

He pushes her forward for their appraisal. "This is Wendy."

Her wet cotton nightgown sticks to her body. It clings to her legs, is plastered to the hollow of her navel and sucked into the indentation of her belly button. But it's the outline of her nipples, stiff with large aureole that are unexpected on such a petite young girl, that make every boy there go hard. From the look in her eyes, they know she's too stunned by the flight to realize this. From Peter's lascivious grin, they know he flew her through a rainfall on purpose.

"Say hi," he urges, dropping his hand to gently cup her ass.

She blushes deeply. "Um . . . hello."

No one says a word. The boys stare at her with a grim and begrudging lust. Then Peter flashes a cocky smile at his tribe and says, "Be back soon" and leads Wendy away into the night.

Concealed behind her rock, Tigerlily watches, scarcely daring to breathe as Peter saunters confidently to a banyan tree and tugs Wendy next to him. "Sorry I got you wet," he murmurs and kisses her ear, but not before another smug and secret grin escapes him at his own wordplay. Wendy doesn't notice it but only because she's growing suspicious now; she's looking uncertain of this long-limbed devil who shimmied up her drainpipe and crept through her bedroom window. That had to be how he did it, Tigerlily thinks, his naughty grin appearing at the window like every repressed fantasy of her good girl imagination. For Wendy is definitely a good girl, procured by him in some hushed fancy place full of manicured gardens and teatime and other things Tigerlily doesn't understand; that's Peter's secret type. Well bred and easily awed and secretly burning to break out of the nursery. Instead the devil came to the nursery. Of course she let him in.

Wendy shivers now with some theatrics, prompting Peter to go predictable: "Are you cold? I'll warm you up."

So boring, so clichéd, Tigerlily thinks, she should interrupt and teach them a thing or two. Still she wants to see Wendy's nightgown come off and that is exactly what happens, as Peter's mouth moves across her throat so skillfully that his hands push the nightgown up her hips without notice. Up it rises to reveal oval knees and soft pale legs. Something stirs deep in Tigerlily's body. Moments later, Wendy's cunt comes into view, a soft mound of hair that doesn't quite conceal her shy cleft. Then her hips, rather wide and narrowing up into her waist, and finally her tits, full and round and creamy with those pink saucerlike nipples. Perfect breasts, the kind Tigerlily wants to feel bouncing against her own as the two of them fuck each other into oblivion.

She drags her gaze up to check Wendy's face. The girl is scarlet with embarrassment and trembling. She should be spanked, Tigerlily thinks, turned over my knee and spanked until her creamy ass is as red as her face. Then she'll cry and I'll lick her tears away . . .

Wendy's body is so pale and soft. This is a naked body that has never seen sunlight, Tigerlily can tell, and this is a girl who has never felt a man's touch anywhere beneath the neck. That's clear as Peter, too fascinated to bother with sexual amenities now, traces one finger over her slit. Wendy's legs open and her eyes close with shame. "Oh my God," she whispers.

Tigerlily's blood grows hot. She cannot bear to watch this a moment longer, Peter with yet another girl, so soft and obedient. In moments he will be playing with her clit and stroking the insides of her pussy until what will possibly be the girl's first orgasm slams through her—and then those soft doe eyes will gaze at him in a way no girl has ever gazed at *her* . . .

She scrambles silently through the trees, scales one, and launches into her best pirate voice. The warning she calls out is ridiculous—Peter would be stupid to react to it so immediately; they played Pirate a dozen times together as kids, but his lust for war is stronger than his tactician's instincts and he abandons Wendy in a second. "Wait here!" he commands, all boy-man authority, and fairly skips off to the Lost Boys, his boys, who are already creeping toward battle.

Such an idiot, Tigerlily thinks. Always forsaking the girl for the adventure—that's Peter. But no mind. She runs back through the trees and is at Wendy's side before the girl can put her nightgown back on.

Wendy is sure she is going to be murdered. The girl looming over her is like no girl she's ever seen, barely clad in a tiny buckskin dress, her long black hair alive in the night wind. Even her voice is different and commanding as she hisses, "Shut up! I'm Tigerlily; I'm a friend of Peter's. The pirates are here, I'm going to rescue you." At the word *pirates*, something blank and primitive tightens Wendy's throat and she can't say a word as the girl snatches down the nightgown from its branch and ties the sleeve quickly and expertly in a gag through her pretty mouth. Wendy chokes a bit but she has been gagged before in her brothers' games and perhaps that is why she doesn't protest as the black-haired girl ties up her wrists with the other sleeve and leads her off into the forest.

Or perhaps she doesn't protest because of the cumulative shock of the night, which began tossing restlessly in her bed: too old at eighteen to spend her nights staring at the London rooftops through the nursery window. There was the shock of seeing a beautiful boy her own age appear at the window with a devilish smile, a boy who climbed in to shamelessly appraise her body through the skimpy nightgown before taking her hand and tugging her out the window. The shock of flying away over London, the shock of being stripped naked and spreading her legs as Peter touched her pussy. And now this, being tied up and led off into the woods, a naked captive. Not captured by a man like in her most forbidden fantasies but by a girl—a girl with hard lean muscles and long legs who moves so fast Wendy stumbles behind her.

Dazed as she is, it takes a minute to replay Tigerlily's words and realize their basic contradiction: that if Tigerlily is Peter's friend, why did she tie Wendy up? Her bare feet hurt from the sticks and debris of the jungle floor and the night chill is making her stiff nipples ache. No one knows where she is. Yet soon enough they stop in a clearing, where Tigerlily pushes her to her knees before building a fire. She stockpiles a supply of kindling, then takes her place opposite the flames.

Now the two girls stare at each other. Wendy can see every detail of her kidnapper's face in the firelight: a fiercely beautiful girl a little older than her with high cheekbones and fiery eyes, and a tough mouth that Wendy can tell will know exactly what to do to her. Everything about her wiry, taut body screams of sexual knowledge. This is a girl who knows what to do.

Then Tigerlily drops her eyes and draws all that glorious black hair over one shoulder as she gazes into the fire. She seems absentminded, tracing a bruise on one bare thigh—and it is following the movement of her hand that Wendy realizes Tigerlily's legs are slightly open and her pussy is on full display. She seems either unaware of this or indifferent.

Wendy swallows nervously. She has never seen another woman's pussy, has never even gotten a good look at her own. She stares at it now, its mysterious pink folds, and wonders exactly where Peter had touched her to make that electric feeling ring through her.

Tigerlily looks up, notices her gaze and smirks. Wendy swallows again but doesn't remove her eyes. Yet Tigerlily bounces abruptly to her feet, ending the show, and is at her side with that terrifying swiftness again. Roughly she pulls the knotted nightgown sleeve from her mouth. "Sorry."

Wendy's tongue, dry and stiff and tasting of cotton, moves tentatively around her mouth. Her knees hurt and Tigerlily seems especially tall standing before her. "Who—why did you bring me here?"

"Why did Peter bring you to Neverland?" Tigerlily is staring down at her with blank obsidian eyes, but Wendy can tell from the humming tension of her body that she is feeling far from blank at the moment.

"I—I don't know."

"He brought you here to fuck you, Wendy." Tigerlily yanks the nightgown still tied around her hands and brings her roughly to her feet. Then she jerks Wendy's arms up over her head and moves her back and forth like a marionette, making her breasts bounce and sway.

Fear and arousal set off a throbbing between Wendy's legs. No one has ever taken such blatant control of her nor treated her so rudely, and it's exciting. As Tigerlily pushes her back toward a tree, she finds herself turning up her face expectantly for the other girl's mouth. Instead, Tigerlily ropes the knotted nightgown on a branch, imprisoning Wendy's arms over her head. With a dirty smirk, she takes both her tits in her hands and begins to play with them.

"I bet you went to boarding school," Tigerlily accuses.

"I did . . . "

"And I bet all you girls got in each other's beds at night."

"No! No, I mean, some girls, yes . . . "

"But not you?"

"No." Wendy shakes her head too fervently, her damp brown hair falling over her nipples. Tigerlily impatiently flings the hair away, then slaps her breasts hard as punishment.

"You don't cover yourself around me." She pinches her right nipple, making Wendy gasp. "Understand?"

"Yes." That excitement in her pussy feels like melting honey now. Soon her thighs will be wet with it and Tigerlily will see it and then she'll really be punished.

"So." Tigerlily resumes feeling her tits, almost in a detached exploratory manner. "You never wanted a girl to do things to you?"

"Well, I . . . " Wendy can't say the truth of this, which is that the shadow who tops her in her fantasies never has a face, let alone a gender. The shadow only has hands that stroke her, a tongue that licks her, a heat that's sometimes as hard as the hardest cock and other times pillowy as the softest breasts.

"Yes or no, Wendy. It's not that difficult a question."

"Leave her alone."

The rising heat cools in Wendy as she turns to see Peter in the clearing. He's here to rescue her, she realizes with a pang of annoyance, but she's not quite ready to be rescued. His mouth is set in a hard little line, but those green eyes aren't quite as angry as his voice pretends. Yes, he's pissed that Tigerlily stole his prey—his catch, Wendy thinks—but watching her tied up naked as Tigerlily flicks at her nipples isn't something he's ready to stop just yet.

"You're the one who took her out of her own bed and flew her here, Peter," Tigerlily taunts him. "Shouldn't *you* have left her alone?"

She smacks Wendy's breasts together a few times as if they're balloons, then dips her fingers between her legs. "Spread," she orders. Wendy's face burns hot now as she obeys, thighs shaking with anticipation of that first penetration of Tigerlily's fingers. But Tigerlily only traces one light finger around her clit in a soft, maddening circle without taking her eyes from Peter. I am just a pawn to her, Wendy thinks. The thought only makes her clit harder.

"Come on, Peter," Tigerlily smiles. "Come rescue your pet."

So he's here at last. Peter looks as confused as Tigerlily has ever seen him look, rubbing his hair in a way he does when he's thinking. It's rumpled around his face like a golden-red halo, as if he's an angel with a giant cock rather than the arrogant smartass she knows him to be. Once again he's shirtless, his bare chest smooth in the firelight, and two war stripes adorn his sculpted cheekbones. He stopped to paint himself to do battle with the pirates: how ridiculous. Tigerlily gestures to the erection swelling in his pants.

"This is probably a little much for you, so maybe you better just watch."

He flings himself at her with a roar. She dodges him well, with the practice of a hundred mock battles between them, then brings him down on his back. He looks stunned as she straddles him, quickly tying his hands tight with a piece of rope. But he recovers immediately.

"I can bust right out of these knots." He snarls at her in a way that reminds her of defensive animals trying to ward off a predator.

She shifts the heat and pressure of her pussy on his erection. He goes still. Subtly, with a clever smile, she rocks back and forth. His cock swells even bigger until a strangled groan escapes him.

Stupid boy, you don't know what you've been missing, she thinks. But all she says is: "I know what you want." Wendy's impatience and jealousy is palpable by the tree, but Tigerlily ignores her for now. Staring into Peter's eyes, she opens her knees until she's showing him her pussy. So many times she's thought of Peter reaching for her, asking her, begging her, but now she's controlling him and his submission is better than any of her dreams.

"Oh fuck yeah," Peter mutters, his eyes locked on her.

With one quick move she swings up and settles her crotch directly on Peter's mouth. "Do it," she commands, not because he doesn't understand what she wants but because the sound of her own authority arouses her. She is soaked, wet from her clit to her asshole, and she takes pleasure in smearing it all over his nose and eyelids and cheekbones until his arrogant face shines with it.

"Fuck me," Peter moans against her, somewhat illogically as his tongue is desperately seeking her slit. She lifts herself just out of reach to tease him, then relents and sits down on him until the agile heat of his tongue squirms inside her.

Deep euphoria spreads through her. "Just like that," she whispers. She had known this would be good, but just the sight of his face framed between her thighs sends an electric power through her body. Peter's endlessly talking tongue finally silenced and fucking deep in her pussy at last, his wrists tied so he can't fly. This is her moment.

Tigerlily reverses direction on his face, leans over and takes off his pants. Then the prize is in her hands at last: Peter's hard and straining cock. She rolls his shaft between her hands for only a moment before sucking it into her mouth, all of it, until her nose is buried in his balls. He tastes mustier than she expected, a boyish earthy taste, and his cock is as alive in her mouth as an animal. She pulls back to suck his head hard, tonguing it until he gasps.

Peter's not licking her pussy anymore; his tongue has slid up to frantically push inside her asshole, spearing her tightness over and over. And it's this that really does it for her: the knowledge of his tongue in her ass pushes her over into complete orgasmic mindlessness. Her pussy squeezes over and over as a hot gush of ejaculate floods out of her. Beneath her, he pulls back in surprise but she sits down on his face and rides out her orgasm, grinding against his mouth until the last waves sputter out.

His hips bang the ground in frustration. "Tiger—"

She doesn't bother silencing him. Instead, she returns to his cock, pressing it flat against his belly and wiggling her tongue up and down and around him before sucking him back inside her mouth. He writhes beneath her as if he's gone mad. "Don't—oh god—don't stop." She keeps sucking him, feeling his balls tighten right up until the moment of no return—and then she does stop, because after making her wait for so many years, Peter really has no right to any kind of satisfaction this early in the night.

He sinks his teeth into the right cheek of her ass with a long, frustrated groan.

Oh, you *bastard*, she thinks with a mixture of indignation and amusement. She reaches back and feels the bite mark on her ass. Her fingers come away tinged with blood.

"You little bitch," she says and rings him across the face. It only turns him on more, making his hips dance. Her fingertip traces the bite again. Sometime tomorrow she will hold a mirror before her lifted legs and stare at the teeth marks as she fingers herself. But for now she feigns outrage.

"Get up." She yanks him to his feet, a naked and dazed boy looking almost sick with lust. His cock strains toward her as if magnetized. She shoves him against the tree and ropes him next to Wendy. Then she turns their bodies toward each other and begins to play with them like dolls. First she brushes Wendy's nipples against his chest until her face burns tomato-red. Then she strokes Peter's cock over Wendy's slit, pressing his head hard against her clit until they both moan.

Tigerlily laughs. "It's not going to be that easy."

She returns them to their separate positions and begins to toy with them. They look so beautiful, so flushed and horny. Sliding her fingers deep into Wendy's wet and swollen cunt, she rubs her in the way she likes herself, pressing her knuckles against the walls of her pussy. Wendy's pale body steams and shakes, she twists against her bonds and begs to be fucked.

Tigerlily pulls out to stroke her clit. "Is this what you want?"

Wendy's legs strain open. "No . . . !"

"Tell me what you want."

"Just fuck me," Wendy gasps, a pink flush spreading across her breasts. She seeks to bring Tigerlily closer by locking her ankles around her but Tigerlily deftly steps out of her way. "Don't stop, oh, please don't."

She fingers Wendy's clit for a few moments longer, then slides in three fingers, deep as she can go. Now she fucks her hard and rapidly, holding Wendy around the waist so she has to take it. Her cunt feels impossibly full and wet around her fingers and as a low growl breaks from her mouth, Tigerlily feels her come; Wendy's velvety heat clenches her over and over until wet aftershocks tremble deep in her own pussy.

Tigerlily gently withdraws her fingers and smears the glistening juices over Peter's parted lips. His eyes are locked on her, not Wendy, with reverence. Oh Peter, she thinks, we haven't even started.

"Kiss me," she says. Her mouth, her tough mouth that has insulted and mocked him so many nights and cried his name alone in her bedroom, covers his. He tastes of Wendy's honeyed brine and then his own surprising sweetness. A sweet boy with a hard cock, captured at last. He's not flying anywhere until she's done with him, and the night has only begun as she presses her cool long body against his flushed and trembling one. Tigerlily twists her arms up around his neck like a lover, like she dreamed of when she was young and romantic and naive. But now she grabs his thick soft hair in her fist and twists it, pulling his head back so she can bite his lips.

"Anything you want," he begs in a low voice. "But please, please . . . "

What I want, she thinks, is to fly. And then it's happening, his cock pushes into the initial tightness of her pussy, demanding and inexorable yet torturously slow. She hooks one leg around his waist and brings him in deeper inch by teasing inch, until the cool sack of his balls rests against her. Already she's beginning to throb as they start to thrust, his heat and his hardness driving her up and up into blinding wet bliss, and then they're really fucking, faster and faster until at last Tigerlily is flying.

VALERIE ALEXANDER is a freelance writer who lives in Arizona. Her work has been previously published in *Best Lesbian Erotica*, *Best of Best Women's Erotica*, and other anthologies.

LET G BE YOUR GUIDE

If you're a G-spot or female ejaculation beginner, I hope this book has opened up a new world of sexual possibilities for you, including plenty of novel things to explore.

Experimenting with new techniques can help diversify your masturbation routine or the sex you have with your partner or, ideally, both. Even if you have plenty of sexual experience, there's no time like the present to try something different, teach yourself some new tricks, and expand your horizons. G-spotting and learning to ejaculate can intensify the pleasure and orgasms you already have. If you're someone who has trouble having an orgasm during vaginal intercourse, homing in on the G-spot may be a way for you to enjoy it more and even climax from it. It's also a great excuse to buy a new sex toy! If you've tried G-spot stimulation and female ejaculation before, I hope this validates your experiences and gives you some information to make it even better.

Spread the word about what you learn in this book to other women. Information about the G-spot and female ejaculation should no longer be a *secret*. We need to have more information sharing and fewer mysteries about our sexuality. Every woman has a right to know about her anatomy, pleasure, and orgasm—her full sexual potential.

Every woman has a urethral sponge and the area on the front wall of the vagina that butts up against it, so every woman has a G-spot. The way women experience G-spot stimulation is what is so varied—it may do nothing for you, it may create unique sensations, it may just feel really good, it may give you knock-your-socks-off orgasms, or it may make you squirt.

Discovering your G-spot is not about reaching for some specific goal. Don't try G-spot stimulation or female ejaculation because you think it's the cool new thing to do, the key to the best sex of your life, or what your partner wants. Don't load yourself down with unrealistic expectations or put pressure on yourself. Remember, it's all about the journey: exploring the wonders of your body, discovering new erogenous zones and different kinds of stimulation, and embracing your sexual potential. As you wander through this new territory, be patient, give yourself time, and don't expect orgasmic lightning to strike in the beginning. Do it because it feels good. Do it because you want to. Do it for you.

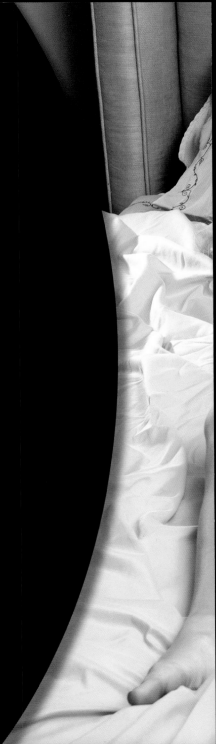

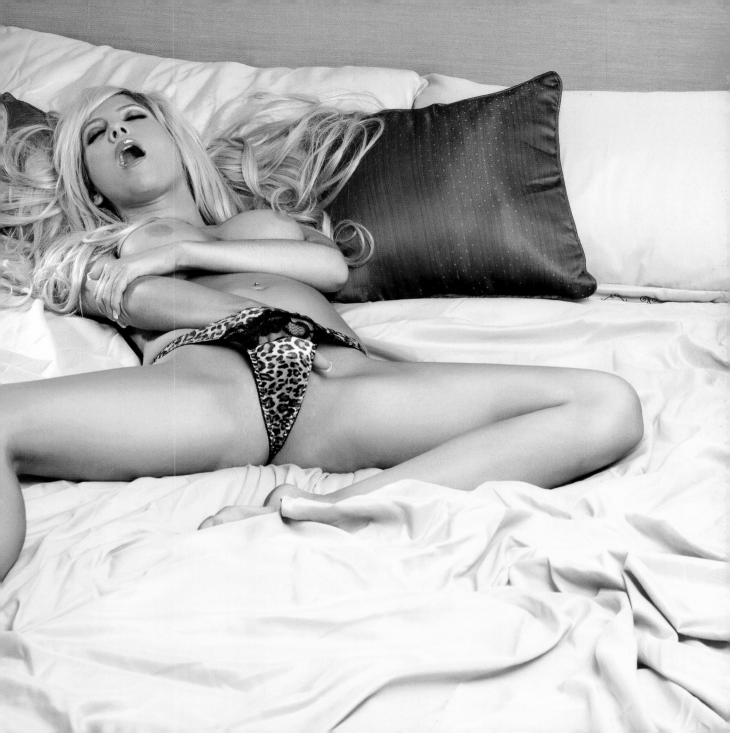

RESOURCE GUIDE

BOOKS

The Anal Sex Position Guide by Tristan Taormino. Beverly, MA: Quiver Books, 2009.

The Big Book of Sex Toys by Tristan Taormino. Beverly, MA: Quiver Books, 2010.

The Clitoral Truth: The Secret World at Your Fingertips by Rebecca Chalker. New York: Seven Stories Press, 2003.

Dr. Sprinkle's Spectacular Sex: Make Over Your Love Life with One of the World's Great Sex Experts by Annie Sprinkle. New York: Tarcher/Penguin, 2005.

Female Ejaculation and the G-Spot: Not Your Mother's Orgasm Book! by Deborah Sundahl. Alameda, CA: Hunter House, 2003.

The Good Vibrations Guide to Sex: The Most Complete Sex Manual Ever Written by Cathy Winks and Anne Semans. San Francisco: Cleis Press, 2002.

The G-Spot: And Other Discoveries About Human Sexuality by Alice Kahn Ladas, Beverly Whipple, and John D. Perry. 2nd ed. New York: Owl Books/Henry Holt and Co., 2009.

Guide to Getting It On by Paul Joannides. 5th ed. Waldport, OR: Goofy Foot Press, 2006.

Healing Sex: A Mind-Body Approach to Healing Sexual Trauma by Staci Haines. San Francisco: Cleis Press, 2007.

I Love Female Orgasm: An Extraordinary Orgasm Guide by Dorian Solot and Marshall Miller. Cambridge, MA: Da Capo Press, 2007.

Nina Hartley's Guide to Total Sex by Nina Hartley with I. S. Levine. New York: Avery, 2006.

The Smart Girl's Guide to the G-Spot by Violet Blue. San Francisco: Cleis Press, 2007.

The Ultimate Guide to Anal Sex for Women by Tristan Taormino. 2nd ed. San Francisco: Cleis Press, 2006.

SEX EDUCATION VIDEOS

The Amazing G-Spot and Female Ejaculation. Directed by Dr. Perry. Los Angeles: Access Instructional Media, 2006.

The Art of Female Ejaculation. HolisticWisdom.com, 2005.

The Expert Guide to Anal Sex. Directed by Tristan Taormino. Vivid-Ed, 2007.

The Expert Guide to Female Ejaculation. Directed by Tristan Taormino. Vivid-Ed, 2011.

The Expert Guide to the G-Spot. Directed by Tristan Taormino. Vivid-Ed, 2008.

Female Ejaculation for Couples. Directed by Deborah Sundahl. Isis Media, 2004.

The G-Spot and Female Ejaculation. Alexander Institute, 2007.

How to Female Ejaculate. Directed by Deborah Sundahl. Isis Media, 1992.

Liquid Love: The G-Spot Explosion. Directed by Godfrey Silas and Leila Swan. Glamour Television, 2006.

Maximizing G-Spot Pleasures. Hillsborough, NC: Sinclair Intimacy Institute, 2007.

Nina Hartley's Guide to Female Ejaculation. Directed by Ernest Greene. Carrboro, NC: Adam & Eve, 2006.

Nina Hartley's Guide to G-Spot Sex. Directed by Ernest Greene. Carrboro, NC: Adam & Eve, 2005.

Tantric Journey to Female Orgasm. Directed by Deborah Sundahl. Isis Media, 1998.

Unlocking the Secrets of the G-Spot. Hillsborough, NC: Sinclair Intimacy Institute, 2000.

STORES

Here is a selection of sex-positive retail stores that sell sex toys.
Many are women-owned and -run and host sex education workshops
on a variety of topics (including the G-spot and female ejaculation);
all are women- and couples-friendly.

A Little More Interesting
alittlemoreinteresting.com
1501B 17th Avenue SW
Calgary, AB
Canada T2T 0E2
403-475-7775

Aphrodite's Toy Box
aphroditestoybox.com
3040 N. Decatur Road
Scottdale, GA 30079
404-292-9700

Art of Loving
artofloving.ca
1819 West Fifth Avenue
Vancouver, BC
Canada V6J 1P5
604-742-9988

A Woman's Touch
a-womans-touch.com
888-621-8880

600 Williamson Street
Madison, WI 53703
608-250-1928

200 N. Jefferson Street
Milwaukee, WI 53202
414-221-0400

Babeland
babeland.com
800-658-9119

707 East Pike Street
Seattle, WA 98122
206-328-2914

94 Rivington Street
New York, NY 10002
212-375-1701

43 Mercer Street
New York, NY 10013
212-966-2120

462 Bergen Street
Brooklyn, NY 11217
718-638-3820

Coco de Mer
Coco-de-mer.com

23 Monmouth Street
London WC2H 9DD
+44 (0)20 7836 8882

108 Draycott Avenue
London SW3 3AE
+44 (0)20 7584 7615

Come As You Are
comeasyouare.com
701 Queen Street West
Toronto, ON
Canada M6J 1E6
888-504-7934

Early to Bed
early2bed.com
5232 N. Sheridan Road
Chicago, IL 60640
866-585-2233

Eros Boutique
erosboutique.com
581A Tremont Street
Boston, MA 02118
866-425-0345

Fascinations
funlove.com
866-FUN-LOVE
Stores in Arizona, Colorado, and Oregon
See website for locations

Forbidden Fruit
forbiddenfruit.com
512 Neches Street
Austin, TX 78701
512-478-8358

108 E. North Loop Boulevard
Austin, TX 78751
512-453-8090

Good for Her
goodforher.com
175 Harbord Street
Toronto, ON
Canada M5S 1H3
416-588-0900

Good Vibrations
goodvibes.com
800-289-8423

603 Valencia Street
San Francisco, CA 94110
415-522-5460

1620 Polk Street
San Francisco, CA 94109
415-345-0400

2504 San Pablo Avenue
Berkeley, CA 94702
510-841-8987

308A Harvard Street
Brookline, MA 02446
617-264-4400

It's My Pleasure
itsmypleasurepdx.com
3106 NE 64th Avenue
Portland, OR 97213
503-280-8080

Nomia Boutique
nomiaboutique.com
24 Exchange Street, Suite 215
Portland, ME 04101
207-773-4774

Oh My: A Sensuality Shop
ohmysensuality.com
122 Main Street
Northampton, MA 01060
413-584-9669

Passional Toys
passional.net
704 S. 5th Street
Philadelphia, PA 19147
877-U-CORSET

The Pleasure Chest
pleasurechest.com
800-753-4536

156 Seventh Avenue South
New York, NY 10014
212-242-2158

3436 North Lincoln Avenue
Chicago, IL 60657
773-525-7151

7733 Santa Monica Boulevard
West Hollywood, CA 90046
323-650-1022

The Rubber Rose
therubberrose.com
3812 Ray Street
San Diego, CA 92104
619-296-7673

Self Serve
selfservetoys.com
3904B Central Avenue SE
Albuquerque, NM 87108
505-265-5815

She Bop
shebopthehsop.com
909 North Beech Street
Portland, OR 97227-1258
503-473-8018

Smitten Kitten
smittenkittenonline.com
3010 Lyndale Avenue South
Minneapolis, MN 55408
612-721-6088

Spartacus
spartacusstore.com
300 SW 12th Avenue
Portland, OR 97205
503-224-2604

The Stockroom
stockroom.com
2807 W. Sunset Boulevard
Los Angeles, CA 90026
800-755-8697

Sugar
sugartheshop.com
927 W. 36th Street
Baltimore, MD 21211
410-467-2632

The Tool Shed

toolshedtoys.com
2427 N. Murray Avenue
Milwaukee, WI 53211
414-906-5304

Tulip Toy Gallery

mytulip.com
877-70-TULIP
1480 W. Berwyn Avenue
Chicago, IL 60640
773-275-6110

3459 North Halstead
Chicago, IL 60657
773-975-1515

1422 North Milwaukee Avenue
Chicago, IL 60622
877-70-TULIP

Venus Envy

venusenvy.ca

1598 Barrington Street
Halifax, NS
Canada B3J 1Z6
902-422-0004

320 Lisgar Street
Ottawa, ON
Canada K2P 0E2
613-789-4646

Womyns' Ware

womynsware.com
896 Commercial Drive
Vancouver, BC
Canada V5L 3Y5
604-254-2543

BIBLIOGRAPHY

Belzer, Edwin, Beverly Whipple, and William Moger. "On Female Ejaculation." *The Journal of Sex Research* vol. 20 (1984): 403–406.

Boynton, Petra. "Where Have All the G-Spots Gone?" *Dr. Petra Boynton* (blog) January 4, 2010. www.drpetra.co.uk/blog/where-have-all-the-g-spots-gone.

Burri, Andrea Virginia, Lynn Cherkas, and Timothy D. Spector. "Genetic and Environmental Influences on Self-Reported G-Spots in Women: A Twin Study." *The Journal of Sexual Medicine* vol. 7, no. 5 (2010): 1842–52.

Chalker, Rebecca. *The Clitoral Truth: The Secret World at Your Fingertips.* New York: Seven Stories Press, 2003.

D'Amati, Giulia, Cira di Gioia, Laura Proietti Pannunzi, Daniela Pistilli, Eleonora Carosa, Andrea Lenzi, and Emmanuelle A. Jannini. "Functional Anatomy of the Human Vagina." *Journal of Endocrinological Investigation* vol. 26, suppl. 3 (2003): S92–96.

Davidson, J. Kenneth, Carol A. Darling, and Colleen Conway-Welch. "The Role of the Grafenberg Spot and Female Ejaculation in the Female Orgasmic Response: An Empirical Analysis." *Journal of Sex and Marital Therapy* vol. 15, no. 2 (Summer 1989): 102–20.

The Federation of Feminist Women's Health Centers. *A New View of a Woman's Body.* 3rd ed. Los Angeles: Feminist Health Press, 1995.

Gilliland, Amy L. "Women's Experiences of Female Ejaculation." *Sexuality & Culture* vol. 13, no. 3 (2009): 121–34.

Grafenberg, Ernest. "*The Role of Urethra in Female Orgasm.*" *International Journal of Sexology* vol. 3 (1950): 145–48.

Gravini, Giovanni Luca, Fulvia Brandetti Paolo Martini, Eleonora Carosa, Savino M. Di Stasi, Susanna Morano, Andrea Lenzi, and Emmanuele A. Jannini. "Measurement of the Thickness of the Urethrovaginal Space in Women with or without Vaginal Orgasm." *The Journal of Sexual Medicine* vol. 5, no. 3 (March 2008): 610–18.

Hines, Terence M. "The G-Spot: A Modern Gynecologic Myth." *American Journal of Obstetrics and Gynecology* vol. 185, no. 2 (August 2001): 359–62.

Jannini, Emmanuelle A., Giulia D'Amati, and Andrea Lenzi. "Histology and Immunohistochemical Studies of Female Genital Tissue." In *Women's Sexual Function and Dysfunction: Study, Diagnosis and Treatment*, edited by Irwin Goldstein, Cindy M. Meston, Susan Davis, and Abdulmaged Traish, 125–33. New York: Taylor & Francis, 2006.

Jannini, Emmanuele A., Beverly Whipple, Sheryl A. Kingsberg, Odile Buisson, Pierre Foldès, and Yoram Vardi. "Who's Afraid of the G-Spot?" *The Journal of Sexual Medicine* vol. 7, no. 1 (2010): 25–34.

Kinsey, Alfred C., Wardell C. Pomeroy, Clyde E. Martin, and Paul H. Gebhard. *Sexual Behavior in the Human Female*. Philadelphia: W. B. Saunders, 1953.

Komisaruk, Barry R., C. Beyer, and Beverly Whipple. *The Science of Orgasm*. Baltimore: Johns Hopkins Press, 2006.

Ladas, Alice Kahn, Beverly Whipple, and John D. Perry. *The G-Spot: And Other Discoveries About Human Sexuality*. 2nd ed. New York: Henry Holt and Company, 2009.

Leiblum, Sandra R., and Rachel Needle. "Female Ejaculation: Fact or Fiction." *Current Sexual Health Reports* vol. 3, no. 2 (2006): 85–88.

Masters, William H., and Virginia E. Johnson. *Human Sexual Response*. 4th edition. New York: Little, Brown & Company, 1980.

Masters, William H., Virginia E. Johnson, and Robert C. Kolodny. *Masters and Johnson on Sex and Human Loving*. 4th ed. New York: Little, Brown & Company, 1988.

O'Connell, Helen E., Kalavampara V. Sanjeevan, and John M. Hutson. "Anatomy of the Clitoris." *The Journal of Urology* vol. 174, no. 4 (October 2005): 1189–95.

Perry, John D. "Revised by the Author: A Side-by-Side Comparison of Two Versions of 'The Role of Urethra in Female Orgasm' by Ernest Gräfenberg, M.D." Last modified September 1996. www.incontinet.com/revbyaut.htm.

Singer, Irving. *The Goals of Human Sexuality*. New York: Norton, 1973.

Singer, Irving, and Josephine Singer. "Types of Female Orgasm." *The Journal of Sex Research* vol. 8, no. 4 (November 1972): 255–67.

Sundahl, Deborah. *Female Ejaculation and the G-Spot*. Alameda, CA: Hunter House, 2003.

Whipple, Beverly, and Barry R. Komisaruk. "The G Spot, Vaginal Orgasm, Female Ejaculation: A Review of Research and Literature." In *Sex Matters: Proceedings of the 10th World Congress of Sexology*, edited by Peggy Cohen-Kettenis, Willeke Bezemer, and Koos Slob, 33–36. Amsterdam: Elsevier Science, 1992.

ENDNOTES

1. Elisabeth Anne Lloyd, *The Case of the Female Orgasm: Bias in the Science of Evolution* (Cambridge: Harvard University Press, 2006).

2. Deborah Sundahl, *Female Ejaculation and The G-Spot* (Alameda, CA: Hunter House, 2003), xix.

3. Alice Ladas, Beverly Whipple, and John D. Perry, *The G-Spot and Other Discoveries about Human Sexuality*, 2nd ed. (New York: Henry Holt and Company, 2005), 42.

4. Giovanni Luca Gravini et. al., "Measurement of the Thickness of the Urethrovaginal Space in Women with or without Vaginal Orgasm," *The Journal of Sexual Medicine* vol. 5, no. 3 (March 2008): 610–18.

5. Andrea Burri, Virginia Lynn Cherkas, and Timothy D. Spector, "Genetic and Environmental Influences on Self-Reported G-Spots in Women: A Twin Study," *The Journal of Sexual Medicine* vol. 7, no. 5 (2010).

6. Burri et. al., 1848–49.

7. Tamara Cohen, "'We've Found the G-spot,' Say the French (Of Course)," January 29, 2010, www.dailymail.co.uk/news/article-1246940/Weve-G-spot-say-French-course.html.

8. Epiphora, "My Love, the Pure Wand (+ a Few Tips!)," July 26, 2010, www.heyepiphora.com/2010/07/my-love-the-pure-wand-plus-a-few-tips.

9. Sundahl, 93.

10. Sundahl, 93.

11. Sundahl, 155.

12. Amy L. Gilliland, "Women's Experiences of Female Ejaculation," *Sexuality & Culture* vol. 13, no. 3 (2009): 128.

13. Sandra R. Leiblum and Rachel Needle, "Female Ejaculation: Fact or Fiction," *Current Sexual Health Reports* vol. 3, no. 2 (2006): 85.

14. Milan Zaviacic and Richard J. Albin, "The Female Prostate and Prostate-Specific Antigen, Immunohistochemical Localization, Implications of This Prostate Marker in Women and Reasons for Using the Term 'Prostate' in the Human Female," *Histology and Histopathology* vol. 15, no. 1 (2000): 131–142. F. Cabello, "Female Ejaculation: Myths and Realities" (paper presented at the proceedings of the 13th World Congress of Sexology, June 25–27, 1997, www.drgspot.net/cabello.htm.

15. Gilliland, 122–123.

16. Ladas et. al., 68.

17. Belzer et. al., 1984; Goldberg et. al., 1983; Bullough et. al., 1984; Heath, 1984—all cited in Gilliland, 131.

18. Gilliland, 131.

19. Bonnie Bullough, Madeline David, Beverly Whipple, Joan Dixon et al., "Subjective Reports of Female Orgasmic Expulsion of Fluid," *Nurse Practitioner* vol. 9 (1984): 55–59.

20. Giulia D'Amati et. al., "Functional Anatomy of the Human Vagina," *Journal of Endocrinological Investigation* vol. 26, suppl. 3 (2003): S92–96, and Emmanuelle A. Jannini et. al., "Histology and Immunohistochemical Studies of Female Genital Tissue," in *Women's Sexual Function and Dysfunction: Study, Diagnosis and Treatment*, edited by Irwin Goldstein et. al. (New York: Taylor & Francis, 2006), 125–133.

21. Dr. Susan Block, "It Always Rains in California: All about Female Ejaculation," www.bigozine2.com/features05/SBgspot.html.

22. Sundahl, 52.

23. Sundahl, 51.

24. Cited in Rebecca Chalker, *The Clitoral Truth: The Secret World at Your Fingertips* (New York: Seven Stories Press, 2003), 117.

25. Sundahl, 54.

ABOUT THE AUTHOR

TRISTAN TAORMINO is an award-winning author, columnist, editor, and sex educator. She is the author of seven books, including *The Big Book of Sex Toys*, *The Anal Sex Position Guide*, *Opening Up: A Guide to Creating and Sustaining Open Relationships*, *True Lust: Adventures in Sex*, *Porn and Perversion*, *Down and Dirty Sex Secrets*, and *The Ultimate Guide to Anal Sex for Women,* winner of a Firecracker Book Award. She is series creator and founding editor of eighteen volumes of the Lambda Literary Award-winning anthology *Best Lesbian Erotica*. She runs her own adult film production company, Smart Ass Productions, and is currently an exclusive director for Vivid Entertainment. She directs three series for Vivid: a reality series called *Chemistry*; Vivid-Ed, a sex education series; and *Rough Sex*, a vignette series based around women's real fantasies. She was a syndicated columnist for *The Village Voice* for nine and a half years and writes an advice column for *Taboo* magazine. Tristan and her work have been featured in more than 200 publications including *O: The Oprah Magazine*, *The New York Times*, *Redbook*, *Cosmopolitan*, *Glamour*, *Entertainment Weekly*, *Details*, *New York Magazine*, *Men's Health*, and *Playboy*. She has appeared on CNN, HBO's *Real Sex*, NBC's *The Other Half*, *The Howard Stern Show*, *Loveline*, *Ricki Lake*, MTV, Oxygen, Fox News, The Discovery Channel, and on more than four dozen radio shows. She lectures at top colleges and universities including Yale, Cornell, Princeton, Brown, Columbia, Smith, Vassar, and NYU, where she speaks on gay and lesbian issues, sexuality and gender, and feminism. She teaches sex and relationship workshops around the world, and her official website is tristantaormino.com.